THE GIFT INSIDE

12 STEPS TO HEAL UNWORTHINESS, BROKENNESS AND VICTIM MENTALITY SO YOU CAN FIND YOUR HAPPY

IRINA SHEHOVSOV

CONTENTS

INTRODUCTION

What is it like to wake up and feel grateful?

I often wondered what it would feel like for me to wake up full of gratitude.

When the ground started shaking beneath my feet, I tried to hold on to anything that remained standing.

At that moment I was far from grateful but rather angry, resentful and bitter. I was living in emotional misery, constantly regurgitating the past and recounting the words, thoughts and feelings that kept me firmly stuck right in the muck of it.

I was a prisoner of my own mind. I did not yet know what I didn't know. I dreaded waking up every morning to relive the same reality over again.

This was not the life I imagined, this was not the life I wanted. I often thought of ending my life but the knowing that I was a food provider, aka milk factory for my little one kept me going. I was a robot operating and fulfilling tasks that I thought were required of me. I was an outer shell simply existing, breathing but not feeling alive.

Can you relate?

I found myself recounting all of the mistakes of yesterday, complacency for the sake of acceptance, resentment from a lifetime of feeling used, abused and insignificant, decades of people pleasing and mask wearing.

I wanted to remember the real me.

I remember being called the "smiley Irina" ("Solnyshko") sun which shines so brightly and always smiles, curious about life with many interests and a passion for foreign languages, taking art classes and learning how to tango. I thought life was an exciting and fascinating adventure, I even started writing a novel, but alas never finished it. I had beliefs, values and hopes, the traits that made me who I was.

The upbringing and circumstances of your life often determine how it unfolds, this is what society wants you to believe.

Early on I learnt to be quiet and patient following the slogan of the times, children are to be seen and not heard. Being obedient and silent was encouraged, following rules and never asking why, was adored. Obedient, miss goodie tootsie, people pleaser, the quiet one, never speaking out how I felt, only cared to make others happy, fitting the status quo and playing by their rules.

The fact that I'm now writing this book is a testament that your upbringing doesn't determine the life you create. It's your thoughts that determine your life, the environment where you live, and the people you surround yourself with.

When we are growing up, we imagine a life without worry or trouble. We are taught the conventional: go to school, get good grades, go to college, get a degree, start a career and start a family. Sometimes life throws a curveball and it doesn't come out how we imagined. We are faced with circumstances we think are not of our choosing. But choosing is what we do every day. We say Yes or No, we choose to go or not to go, to be or not to be.

When we choose to do the easy things, life becomes hard. When we do the hard things, life becomes easy. When we honor our values and commitments to self, life becomes easier.

For example, when you choose a partner for the wrong reasons, just so that you are not alone or because everyone around you has someone. Or you are so desperately trying to fit in and be liked everybody else, that you forget that you were once happy, energetic and whole when you were without a partner. You start to merge and blur the lines; you start becoming more like your partner and less like yourself in the process. You no longer recognize who you are. Your personality changes, you blend and change yourself to adapt or comply to make someone else happy. There are no boundaries because you want to be liked and accepted and eventually you forget, you are a person too.

You dismiss the warning signs as you think they're too small to make fuss over. Overtime they add up and little by little you form a different personality. You start to care less. What used to bother you and went against your values, you start to allow, at first with resistance and then slowly but surely it becomes normal.

You learn to dismiss your own worries, to make them small and insignificant. Slowly you begin to feel small and insignificant, and eventually you feel like you are not enough.

You forget how awesome you are, how much you have accomplished and achieved, dreams and desires, values and beliefs, the things you wanted to create. So everyday becomes daunting, a painful reminder and relieving of the past, wondering what you should have said or done differently. You reenact every conversation, thought, and feeling. You turn into a masochist and constantly give yourself a dose of pain and keep yourself firmly stuck in the thoughts of yesterday. You become insane doing the same thing over again and expecting a different result.

Your old life is gone and you feel unable to redefine how to move forward, as you imprison yourself inside the cage of your mind. Living like this is no way to live a life. It is a self-destructing time bomb.

Some people do not see it and get stuck here for their entire lifetime. Living in bitterness all the time. Constantly remembering all the wrongs and ignoring all the rights. These negative thoughts take a heavy emotional toll and often overpower all the positive thoughts.

Did you know that for every "No" you hear, you get to overwrite it with a "Yes", seven times at the minimum. If you are a parent, take a mental note of how often you say No versus Yes to your kid.

Are you hyper focused on perfection?

I'm not suggesting to say yes all the time, but giving praise when something is done good just as much as when mistakes are made.

We are so indoctrinated to focus on negatives, on mistakes and failures, on breaks and misses. Like when the school teacher uses a red pen to highlight everything you got wrong and never recognizes everything you got right.

How does "red ink" show up in your life?

Who reminds you of your failures or says that you're wasting your time?

Is it you or someone in your circle?

The negative is reinforced with emotion and drama, making a physical visceral feeling every time there is a wrong, every time there is a misstep.

Sometimes life is not a straight road and has many twists, turns and stones blocking the way.

Sometimes there are cracks and canyons you have to climb out of.

Sometimes it feels like there are boulders preventing you from moving forward.

These obstacles are unloved pieces of yourself, triggers you may choose to ignore so they keep showing up in your life.

Let's remember that there are always two sides to everything, for every negative there is a positive. There is a lesson to learn, an insight to gain, an opportunity to dig deep and see something from a different perspective.

I learned about a great tool I can use from Mahatria: when a negative event occurs, allow yourself to only speak one sentence about it. When something positive occurs speak three sentences about it. This is to entrain your mind to focus on the positive and to unlearn previous conditioning.

We can't change the past, so there is no sense in upsetting ourselves with the constant reminder. The thinking that created the problem must change to find the solution.

It may be difficult to notice how you're thinking at the moment, but with a little retrospect and the support in this book you can connect the dots.

This book will shed light on how you can reclaim your life.

You already possess everything that you need and my hope is that the tools I share will be instrumental in helping you achieve happiness and fulfillment because it is within your reach.

Use this book as a guide to navigate life after a personal disaster strikes, a loss of a loved one, a loss of identity, a loss of hope, or if you're feeling small and insignificant.

If you feel stuck and are tired of experiencing the same patterns in life.

If you dare to be different and break the status quo, to find your own path and design a life on your terms.

For the women who have spent decades creating a family whilst getting lost in the process. I'm excited to take you on a journey of self-discovery and introduce you to some of the habits that have helped me reshape my life, from a passive observer to an active creator. From a victim of circumstances to a conscious chooser of life experiences and a continuous learner of everything life has to offer.

Every experience, every situation, every circumstance is designed for you to evolve.

Ask yourself:

What do you want to create without any limitations–not bound by time or money?

Who do you want to become, what kind of person and what values do you want to be driven by?

Remember, there is nothing that is impossible. The word itself has "I'm possible" in it!

What follows is my recipe for creating happiness which is found not in the next relationship, next job, next client or new home. It is found right here, right now.

It starts with you!

MORNING ROUTINE

"This being human is a guest house. Every morning a new arrival."

– Rumi

I used to hate my mornings. Waking up to the same reality everyday seemed daunting. Especially when there is nothing to look forward to other than being a milk producer for your newborn. I lived in a fog of uncertainty grasping for something to hold on to. On the outside everything looked "normal", a good job, a home and healthy kids but on the inside I didn't feel normal.

On the inside it felt like the walls were collapsing. The physical pain after having a baby and the emotional pain collided into one deep desire to not want to live anymore. There were days I wondered why I existed, what was the point anyway. Mothering was mostly mechanical, to do what was expected of me, to provide food and shelter. I lived in a home I wanted to run away from and looked for any opportunity to do so. What I didn't realize was no matter how far I ran, I still took myself with me. All the thoughts, feelings and emotions, residue of past traumas, unprocessed grief, sadness and an uncertainty about the future.

Physically, I recovered much faster after my second pregnancy. A week after giving birth, the older one was due to go to kindergarten and off I went getting her there. I strived to get in better shape. I gained less weight with my second pregnancy in fact, you couldn't even tell I was pregnant if looking from behind. Mentally and emotionally, I wasn't really there. I checked out, and didn't feel like I was living. I tried to balance and separate myself in two, to keep one part of me happy for my baby so I wouldn't lose breast milk while the other part of me was suffering in agonizing pain.

I felt like my internal compass was broken. What was considered "normal" no longer made sense. I was seeking what normal looked like and wasn't really finding it anywhere in my immediate surroundings My relationships were shifting and all my married friends were dropping like flies. During the marriage, my partner was the social one who maintained all the external connections. Organizing all the outings and get togethers, I was like an external appendage that came along for the ride. Being an introvert, I didn't need others' company to be entertained. So, I didn't work on maintaining sustainable relationships. The friends I went to school with also had their own families and we saw each other once or twice per year for someone's birthday. There was nothing to look forward to anymore, it felt like life as I knew it was over and I had so many unanswered questions.

How would I be a mom and dad for two children?

I didn't have enough energy to carry me through the day between dropping kids off in two places and then rushing to catch the train. I felt like my best self went to work and my kids would get the leftovers.

So I decided to make some changes.

My first decision was to bring energy back into my life and I started walking in the mornings.

I began my day with a good morning routine and you can too.

Why do you need one, you might ask?

If a routine doesn't sound all that exciting, you probably haven't discovered a good one yet, that is why you think this way. We are creatures of habit.

Did you know 95% of the thoughts you think are exactly the same thoughts that you thought of yesterday?

That's right, only 5% are new.

Given the fact that the average mind is calibrated to the negative, it makes it worse because you keep programming your mind with un-resourceful things. Now add to that your unhealthy surroundings, along with other people who are also dialed in on the negative, and you've got yourself a ticking time-bomb. If you like to check this theory, take a mental note and become an observer of your thoughts instead of being an active participant. Pretty soon you'll discover there is truth to that.

To uninstall faulty software you have to give your mind something new to dwell on. Garbage in, garbage out.

Let's start by tilling the soil. Changes are found in small daily steps that in the long run make your life feel better.

Remember earlier I mentioned, if we choose to do the easy things, life becomes hard.

Change is the only constant in life, yet it is so difficult to change yourself, why is that?

When we are young we have a parent to commandeer us to do the right thing. When we get older it is up to us to make ourselves do the hard things. It is not a natural ability, as we're going against our mind's primary directive, which is to preserve, protect and keep the body safe. Change is a counter to that, it is seen as new, therefore dangerous and must be avoided at all costs.

Our job is to make the uncomfortable comfortable little by little so our mind doesn't feel threatened into a new uncharted territory of change. Our job is to create a plan of small daily actionable steps to get us over the hump and to the promised land, because where we stand now it isn't easy to see.

Pick one habit that you can do for seven days without skipping. The important aspect here is to start small so that you implement and take action. I find that mornings are the most productive part of the day. The magic hours of 5-8 am. If you are not an early riser, try setting your alarm 30 minutes earlier than normal. It may be uncomfortable at first but it is the road to freedom and recovery.

I wasn't always an early riser. In fact, I would sleep till the last possible moment, and then hurry to get ready for work. Most mornings I was rushing out the door without breakfast, just in time to catch the train to work. I was in a constant state of hurry. I ask to what end, why must we hurry all the time, life is too short anyway, are we rushing to our death and not really living?

Mornings can be slow or fast; it is up to you. But setting aside time to get yourself ready for the day ahead, not just to wash and dress yourself, but to get your mind in order, get your body in order all require time. Just imagine firing on all your cylinders. Not just looking pretty on the outside and feeling shitty on the inside, but feeling good all around.

This is what a good morning routine can do for you.

My routine didn't come together all at once; it took time, effort and consistency to create how it supports me today. You can create one too, the kind that works for you.

Don't be upset by humble beginnings. Rome wasn't built in one day and so it would be silly to expect something extraordinary when you start. Anytime you do something new it will feel uncomfortable at first.

"When you arise in the morning, think of what a precious privilege it is to be alive, to breathe, to think, to enjoy, to love– then make that day count!" — Marcus Aurelius

This is how my morning routine started. I wanted to walk for years, but somehow, was not creating the time to do that for myself. Until one day, I took that first step over the threshold of my home to discover a road on the other side. I started walking 20 – 30 minutes in the morning and slowly increased to one hour. To allow time for walking I needed to adjust my wake up time. I shifted from sleeping till the last minute to setting my alarm clock a bit earlier. Don't get me wrong, getting out of a cozy and warm bed into the cold and crisp morning didn't feel all that great when I started, but it was a ticket to my freedom.

Looking back, the simple act of walking created miracles in my life. On my walks I am waking up my body from slumber and appreciating all the surroundings. The beautiful shades of the morning sky, as it switches from crimson to scarlet to pink. The wind against my face and the scent of pine trees or the breeze of the ocean. On some occasions I would go to the beach to start my day, where I can ground myself, dig my feet into sand and really connect with nature.

Walking meditation can clear your senses, and the clutter out of the mind.

It gives me mental clarity, hope and creates space for possibility. On my walks I witness the day being born as the sun slowly rises from the horizon. That feeling of being present made me feel like I didn't miss anything, I was right there when the day started. Walking and mind clearing will invite you to take on a day feeling whole, not bitter, resentful, sad or upset. When you take time to "come to your senses", you don't feel rushed, and you take the time needed to be truly you.

During walks I like to listen to podcasts, audio books and motivational talks. All of your senses must be flooded with goodness. You are the guardian of your beautiful garden *aka* mind and you must be on the lookout of what you allow in, as garbage in, garbage out.

Secondly, I started speaking life into myself. I learned this from Tony Robbins, using the power hour to envision your life to not only say what you want, but see it and feel it in your body. If you can see it in your mind's eye you can hold it in your hand.

I created a story of what I wanted my life to be and spoke over it daily. It was nine years ago when the dream of becoming a writer was conceived. I also thought about how I wanted to live my life and feel truly alive, and it was through writing books, creating works of art, speaking and singing on stages and traveling the world.

You are a powerful creator, you too can envision your life in this way. Creating what you want instead of taking the cards you've been dealt.

What does your life look like when there are no limitations of time and money?

What does your life look like when you are living your dream?

Life is short and precious but somehow, we think we'll do something we always wanted when it is the right time. There will never be the right time, do what you want to now.

Give it some thought, if you are a parent, were you ready to have children, was the time right? No matter how prepared you think you are, your world will be turned upside down and you will have to expand it to allow for children.

How about that notion that you work in a job until you retire and then you'll do what you want. Youthfulness is wasted on the young, by the time you retire, you'll feel so beaten down by living someone else's life, that you'll check out at the end of it. There are two times when we die, once when we're put in the ground and another time when your spirit is broken or you become so numb that you don't care what is going on around you. Living in pursuit of your dream is what makes life meaningful, it makes one feel alive with hope.

Little by little I was adding on to my daily routine of walking and having a green smoothie.

Journaling came next. I started recording how I felt each day and anything that was on my mind. Journaling is a great tool to have in your tool belt. Unburdening your mind and data dumping are great ways to get thoughts out of your system, I call it, laying it on paper. There is something about putting pen to paper. My ideas flow easily and are expressed freely. I recommend decluttering your mental cabinet.

According to research, we generate 60,000 thoughts per day, and that's a lot. Journaling allows you to free up space in your mind, just like a computer running out of RAM when too many applications are running, your mind can run out of space. It can be simple yet profound. Introspection is a great idea as you discover more about yourself and reflect on your own thinking and being.

The next addition to my routine became exercise and there are plenty to choose from. When I'm short on time I do high intensity workouts (HIIT), designed to get your heart racing in no time. Additionally, yoga, pilates, stretching, swimming, a dance workout or a peaceful warrior routine.

Check out the peaceful warrior routine here: https://www. irinashehovsov.com/tgi

Do something to move your body for 20 minutes or more to get dopamine and endorphins rushing through your blood-stream. Setting aside time in the morning allows you to build and chisel yourself by the habits you employ. You start to show up better for yourself and others. You become more resilient, less reactive and ready to tackle any challenge that comes your way.

Morning is the best time to charge your batteries, increase your energy and focus, and prepare you for anything life throws your way.

Here is a sample morning routine, feel free to adjust your wake up time.

A Sample Morning Routine
5:00 – Wake Up + Bathroom
5:20 – Meditation

5:40 – Glass of Water + Morning Walk

6:00 – Stretching/HIIT/Yoga/Pilates

6:10 – Journaling

6:20 – Reading

6:40 – Doing something you love (singing, baking, painting etc)

7:00 - Breakfast

HEALTHY EATING

"Exercise is king; nutrition is queen. Put them together and you've got a kingdom." – Jack LaLanne

*I*n this chapter, we explore the profound connection between what we consume and how we feel, not just physically but emotionally and mentally as well. Food is more than fuel; it's a form of self-care, a daily opportunity to nurture our body, mind, and spirit. When you eat well, you build a strong foundation that supports every other aspect of your well-being.

There is a lot that can be said about nutrition. The main point that I want you to glean from this chapter is not to have a diet with restrictions but rather to make a lifestyle out of healthy eating. The purpose behind healthy eating is to support you in having a vibrant and vital life full of energy. Your life force depends on it. The food choices you make today impact you and your family. You are what you eat, so make fruit and vegetables your best friend. Substitute sugars by finding natural alternatives. A diet full of leafy greens, nuts and vegetables also promotes great brain function. I am not a doctor or a nutritionist, so I encourage you to consult with them first.

Alcohol is not a good supplement if you want to drown your sorrows. It only lasts a short time and if not handled early can become an addiction. Not to mention it is not good for you.

We also get so distracted by the media, TV and advertisements that promote quick satisfaction, whether it is a sugar craving or nice juicy steak, try to look at the long-term effect before giving into this immediate pleasure.

Everyone can decide for themselves, but choosing a healthy and holistic lifestyle is what helped me recover and create a magnificent journey.

The journey of exploration never stops as you discover new ways of living and being.

Another improvement that inadvertently came into my life was a result of stumbling upon a podcast where a Chemistry PHD professor was describing the process of digestion. I will spare you the details. I was so fascinated and engrossed by it that I stopped eating meat. As a result, I lost 10lbs which was not my intent. I simply wanted to take better care of myself since there was no one to take care of me.

I no longer had a midday fog or craving for a snack, I started getting sick less and improved my well-being. It was interesting as I discovered I could live without meat. I was introduced to many legumes and grains that were usually outside my regular repertoire. I became more adventurous in the kitchen by introducing new dishes and perfecting my cooking skills. I practiced this way of eating for nearly five years. I did start having chicken and fish again in moderation, once or twice a week or at family gatherings. I would not say that I ever had challenges with weight or digestion, I wanted to approach this new way of eating with curiosity and experiment to see the result.

In summer of 2021, I started training to be a holistic coach with a focus on wellness and nutrition. I learned more about a whole food diet, not in a sense of restrictions but rather to make sure whatever I eat is whole, minimally processed and full of vitamins and nutrients. And where fats, proteins and carbohydrates are present in moderation and for good measure.

Whole foods—those that are unprocessed and closest to their natural state—are the cornerstone of a nourishing diet. These foods are rich in vitamins, minerals, and other essential nutrients and they provide the body with everything it needs to function optimally.

Fruits, vegetables, whole grains, nuts, seeds, and lean proteins not only give us energy but also repair and strengthen our cells, boost our immune system and support our mental clarity. Unlike processed foods, which often come loaded with additives, sugars, and unhealthy fats, whole foods are pure, offering a direct connection to nature and the healing properties it provides.

Incorporating more whole foods into your diet doesn't have to be overwhelming. Start by making small, manageable changes —perhaps replacing sugary snacks with a handful of nuts or fresh fruit, or opting for whole grains like brown rice or quinoa over refined options.

Over time, these small changes add up, leading to significant improvements in your overall health and well-being.

During my studies, the concept of Holobowl was introduced, a simple, yet satisfying mouthwatering dish. The bowl was created from a scientific perspective and composed using all the food groups, fats, proteins, complex carbohydrates, etc. It came out aesthetically pleasing and was also good for you. It was simple to prepare and easy to incorporate into weekly meal preparation.

You can check out a recipe here. https://www.irinashehovsov. com/tgi

Listening to your body is key, oftentimes we mistake hunger for thirst. Next time you feel hungry try drinking water instead and see if that solves it. Hydration is an important aspect for wellbeing. It is not just quenching your thirst but hydrating your whole body. Adding a pinch of pink Himalayan salt does exactly that. The benefits of pink Himalayan salt are vast. It promotes better health, improves digestion, and circulation. It can also help reduce stress, improve mood, and even support bone health.

Water is the essence of life, yet its often overlooked in discussions about nutrition. Staying adequately hydrated is crucial for every function in your body. Water aids digestion, helps transport nutrients, regulates body temperature and flushes out toxins. It also plays a critical role in maintaining mental clarity and emotional stability.

Dehydration, even in mild forms, can lead to fatigue, irritability, and difficulty concentrating. It can exacerbate feelings of overwhelm and stress, making it harder to navigate challenging times. That's why making hydration a priority is essential, especially when recovering from a traumatic experience.

Aim to drink at least 8 glasses of water a day, more if you are active or live in a hot climate. You can also boost your hydration by incorporating water-rich foods into your diet, such as cucumbers, melons, oranges, and leafy greens. Herbal teas and broths are also excellent options, providing both hydration and additional nutrients.

"Every time you eat or drink, you are either feeding disease or fighting it."

– *Heather Morgan*

Eating is not just a physical act; it's a sensory experience that can ground us in the present moment. Practicing mindful eating—paying full attention to the taste, texture, and aroma of your food—can transform your relationship with what you eat. It encourages you to slow down, savor each bite, and truly listen to your body's hunger and fullness cues.

When you eat mindfully, you're less likely to overeat or turn to food for emotional comfort. Instead, you begin to see food as a source of nourishment and joy, a way to honor and care for yourself. This practice can be particularly healing for those who have experienced trauma, as it helps to rebuild a sense of trust and safety within the body.

Creating a routine around your meals can provide a sense of stability and comfort, especially when you're feeling lost or out of control. Regular mealtimes help regulate your metabolism, stabilize blood sugar levels, and prevent the energy crashes that can affect your mood and mental state.

Try to plan and prepare your meals ahead of time, ensuring you have healthy options readily available. This not only saves time but also reduces the temptation to reach for quick, unhealthy choices. As you establish a nourishing eating routine, you'll find that your body begins to respond positively, with more energy, better mood, and a greater sense of well-being.

Embracing Food as Medicine

Hippocrates famously said, "Let food be thy medicine and medicine be thy food." This ancient wisdom still holds true today. When we view food as a form of medicine, we begin to see it as a powerful tool for healing and transformation.

Let's explore specific foods that can support your recovery from trauma. For example, leafy greens like spinach and kale are rich in folate, which can help reduce symptoms of depression. Omega-3 fatty acids, found in fish like salmon and in flaxseeds, have been shown to improve mood and cognitive function. Probiotic-rich foods like yogurt and sauerkraut support gut health, which is closely linked to mental health.

By making thoughtful choices about what you eat, you can harness the power of nutrition to support your journey toward happiness and inner peace.

Nourishing yourself through whole foods and proper hydration is an act of self-love. It's a way to honor your body and provide it with the resources it needs to heal, grow, and thrive. As you continue on this journey, remember that it's not about perfection, but about progress and consistency. Each healthy choice you make is a step toward a brighter, more vibrant life.

MOVEMENT

⸎

"Exercise is the key not only to physical health but to peace of mind" – Nelson Mandela

---

*L*ife is movement and movement is life. Our bodies were designed to move. When we do not we send a signal to our brain that it's not an important activity. Our brain is a very efficient processor and will only spend resources on what's important. You always have a choice whether to move or not, where you expend your energy will determine your life experience.

If you don't want to spend time moving, you may lose the ability to be a vibrant, flexible, energetic and excited human being. I have been there not wanting to move and exercise, I am not a gym going person not by far. So dragging myself out of bed in the morning wasn't a pleasant activity. Sometimes we get to do the hard things and life gets easier as a result.

Why would you want to move?

Why is moving important?

There are countless articles on the subject. You are killing two birds with one stone. When you exercise your body you send happy hormones through your system and your self-esteem improves as a result. Little by little you become a different person, one that takes care of their vessel and strives to have the best possible living experience. You become resilient, you get sick less, your body becomes your temple.

Of course, you always have a choice of how you spend your time.

Do you prefer to spend your time getting healthy or would you rather spend it being sick?

Being healthy consists of a daily commitment, it requires intent and taking action.

Being sick does not require any commitment, it just steals away your joy, takes away your aliveness, creates dullness and melancholy.

Which would you rather create?

If you choose a healthy living experience then I invite you to explore the wonderful world of fitness which does not neces- sarily involve trips to the gym, if it is not your forte. I personally do not enjoy the gym, I prefer nature and outdoors. Walking, running, swimming, and dancing is never boring but rather invigorating as you get to energize your senses.

For strength and resistance training I was introduced to an awesome world of 10x training program. I completed my coaching certification and am now able to pass on that lifestyle to others. What attracted me to it wasn't a hit and run solution or a hardcore training workout. I mean it feels intense when you're in it, but it is not a rigorous daily grind in the gym. It is a lifestyle that I enjoy and it encourages me to keep going. A short fifteen minute workout two times per week was all it took to create and maintain my strength training routine. It focuses on major muscle groups and specific targeted exercise routines designed to be effective and efficient. It can be practiced at home or at the gym. I opted for the home workout and purchased a pull-up bar, adjustable dumbbells, a back roller and some resistance bands. That was all I needed.

I surprised myself with that program by also becoming a student of the routines. Whenever you learn something, you first learn it for yourself, the more you do something, you master the skill and then you're able to transfer the knowledge to others. Unlike other programs you track progress with a special body scan that measures the amount of lean muscle versus fat in addition to a few other metrics. That scan is also taken three months later. In addition to scan, workout progress is tracked on a spreadsheet. Nothing shows progress better than when you can see your own results documented over time. I lost fat and gained muscle, but you would not see that on a regular scale that measures your weight. The body scan proved to me the progress I was experiencing and motivated me to go forward.

Other great benefits I experienced were that my lower back pain was gone. The back pain would appear in the morning upon waking up. It was a remnant of epidural application from my son's birth seven years prior. The pain would dissipate by the mid morning. So it was a nice reprieve not having that anymore. My strength has increased and I am fully using my body. The body is a miraculous organism with many systems that guide and regulate. By exercising regularly you create optimal conditions for all systems to function better. Just like a plant that needs good soil, water and sun, exercise creates a fertile soil and one of the building blocks on which a healthy body is built.

Sleep

Physical health wouldn't be complete without sleep. Sleep is an underrated superpower. In a constantly under-slept world, lack of sleep is responsible for sour mood, being out of touch with your body and not feeling alive. Aliveness is the spice of life. Of course there are days when sleep is not the best, but if it is a constant problem then you might want to look into sleep deprivation.

Sleep adds vitality to your day. The quality of your sleep is the direct result of your evening routine. You create the conditions to unwind and then sleep happens as a natural byproduct.

When your days are filled with many juggling balls that give you anxiety, it could be difficult to quiet the overactive mind.

To help you unwind, create a routine to cut out electronic devices, watching the news, and having arguments two hours before bed. Take your last meal of the day four hours before sleep. The natural renewal and rest cannot happen if the body needs to digest food. The process of digestion is long, so make your last meal before sleep light on your system.

If you still feel charged up from the day's activities, do some breathing exercises to help slow your breathing and calm your senses.

Taking a hot shower before bed also helps.

One hour before sleep, prepare your bedroom. Let in some fresh air or turn on your air conditioner. Make the room dark and cold. Invest in some blackout curtains. Charge your phone away in another room, put it in airplane mode or switch to do not disturb. The reason for this is simple, if you find yourself waking up in the middle of the night you have less urge to check your phone.

Finally, when you're tucked into bed, remember your day, recount three things that went well. If you discover more than three, that's good, keep going. The idea here is to retrain your mind to focus on the positive. These could be small things like seeing a smile on your child's face or having that special moment, experiencing something beautiful, or stepping out of your comfort zone and doing something for the very first time. Focusing on the positive doesn't mean that you're avoiding your problems. Simply put, the more you think about your problems, the more problems will come to haunt you. You give life to everything and for your mind it doesn't matter if something is bad or good. It simply executes the command you feed it. The command is a thought that you constantly think or speak about. You might not even notice that you do that, but you do, we all do. We all have the inner narrator constantly measuring, judging and commenting on anything and everything that is happening in and around us. Your job is to feed the narrator empowering messages that are beneficial and make your life better. Remember the same mind that created the problem, can't find the solution by repeating the same and expecting different results, as this is the definition of insanity.

In the morning when you wake up avoid scrolling the phone first thing. Dedicate at least an hour of time to you. Set intentions and goals for the day, wake your body up and fulfill your agenda before you answer the demands of others. Take care of yourself first.

How to add movement to your day

Opt for stairs over elevators. This small choice builds cardiovascular health and leg strength over time.

If you sit all day, set a timer to stand and walk every hour. These short walks keep your energy up and muscles loose.

Incorporate quick stretches throughout the day. A few minutes can ease muscle tension, improve flexibility, and lower injury risk.

Add 1-2 minute bursts of activity like squats or jumping jacks throughout your day. These "exercise snacks" boost circulation, metabolism, and energy, especially when a full workout isn't possible.

Remember, every step you take is a step toward a healthier, more energized version of yourself. It's not about making drastic changes overnight, but embracing small, consistent actions that add up over time. Movement is life, and by adding even a few moments of it to your day, you're nurturing not only your body but also your spirit. So, choose to move— because every choice you make to care for your body is a choice to care for your future.

MEDITATION

"Life is a mystery – mystery of beauty, bliss and divinity.
Meditation is the art of unfolding that mystery." – Amit Ray

*I*n the midst of life's turmoil, when the weight of past traumas bears down, and the future seems uncertain, there lies a profound refuge in the practice of meditation. Meditation, at its core, is about creating space—space to breathe, to reflect, to heal. It is within this stillness that you find motion, a quiet yet powerful movement toward emotional resilience, forgiveness, and gratitude.

Meditation is often perceived as the act of quieting the mind, but in reality, it is an active process of tuning into one's inner world. When someone has experienced trauma, the mind can become a storm of intrusive thoughts, regrets, fears, and anxieties. Meditation offers a safe harbor, a way to anchor oneself amidst these turbulent waters.

Through regular practice, meditation helps to cultivate mindfulness—the ability to observe one's thoughts and emotions without becoming entangled in them. This mindfulness creates a buffer between the self and the trauma, allowing one to process pain and release it rather than holding onto it. Over time, this can lead to profound healing as you learn to let go of the past and focus on the present moment.

My affair with meditation is a recent addition to my daily repertoire. I practice slowing down and coming back to center to tune in to my inner wisdom. Through meditation I have received many answers. When I ask the universe (god) in a form of a prayer, meditation is where I get the answer.

Much of my life was spent rushing to and from, hastily getting ready in the morning, running to catch the train to work. Running from meeting to meeting, then running back home at the end of the day. I had no time to slow down, as I thought my world would fall apart if I did. I realized that slowing down is what was needed to change my life.

Why do I recommend slowing down and being more present?

Because life is fleeting. It's made up of small, tiny moments and when the pace is fast, you miss them. Savoring the moment has proven to increase happiness levels. You can only savor when you are present, not when you are running from place to place or doing busy work to tick the boxes.

The pace of technology has proven to overwhelm the mind giving it no space to rest. What I discovered through slowing down: I am more resilient, I have more energy, I am more present, centered and aware of my surroundings.

Have you ever felt like you are sleepwalking through life, blissfully unaware of what's going on until something happens that doesn't fit the scenario?

Like a piece of a puzzle that doesn't fit?

Meditation aligns your compass of inner knowing, recalibrates your thought patterns into coherent flow. It is like an inner shower for the mind that clears away the debris (cobwebs) of yesterday, arguments, quarrels, misunderstandings. Just like a morning shower makes you feel fresh and smell nice, you want to have fresh thoughts and clear ideas. Meditation is a great tool to support your mental health.

"When things get tough and our bodies start to react, we need mindfulness to reset our internal north star." – George Mumford

---

Sometimes it can be scary to be with your own thoughts. This may be why you distract yourself with phones, movies, conversations, anything not to be alone with your thoughts.

Have you ever noticed that when you listen or watch something, you speed it up, 1.5x or 2x the normal rate? Please tell me I'm not the only one who does this?

Let's talk about creating a space in your life for meditation.

The environment where you meditate matters.

Allocate a space in your home where you can connect to yourself without distractions. Have your favorite pillow and blanket ready. Create a space of serenity and flow. It does not matter when you do this practice, what matters is that you do it consistently.

I found what works best for me is a daily practice in the morning before doing anything else. I charge up my batteries and fill my cup before I become someone for others. My mornings offer me an opportunity to create each day anew, grab a clean canvas and paint my masterpiece.

I start by cleaning out cobwebs from every corner of my mind. Just like cleaning a room, I wipe the dust away. Cleaning your mind of things that adversely affect your life can bring you more peace and joy.

Meditation also helps with the obsession over past hurts. Oftentimes, we live in the past wondering what could have been, what I should have said, how I behaved. The truth of the matter is you cannot change the past, but by perpetuating it in the present, you create more of it for your future. It does not matter for our mind when something happened a decade ago or if something is happening presently. The same parts of the brain light up when we are thinking and feeling those emotions from the past, so we get to feel all those emotions all over again. When this happens, you're sending a signal to your brain that is important, because you are paying attention to that. So, your unconscious mind aka the goal getter will bring what's important to you into your life. You will get confirmation all around you to what you think and feel.

Meditation has been proven to reduce anxiety and depression. It adds clarity and ease to everyday life. You become less reactive to things when you allow your mind to decompress, you become resilient and able to deal with triggering events with grace. Falling asleep becomes easier as well. The benefits are experienced after consistent practice and are not an overnight phenomenon. Come to think of it, everything worthwhile in life requires consistency and practice, masterful execution comes with experience. Don't beat yourself up if you don't get into the groove of things right away. The important thing is to start, as they say, the best time to start was twenty years ago, the next best time is now. The benefits alone are just too good to miss.

Mediation can support you with forgiveness and healing deep levels of trauma.This forgiveness may be directed toward others who have caused harm, or it may be forgiveness of oneself for perceived failures or shortcomings. In meditation, we are invited to sit with our emotions, no matter how painful or uncomfortable they may be. This forgiveness is not a justification of others' wrongdoings. It is forgiveness of self, first and foremost.

We always operate to the best of our ability with the resources we have available at the time. We are not doing it for others, we are doing it for ourselves if we ever want to feel happy again. Dragging heavy emotional baggage takes its toll on your temperament and if left unchecked can manifest in a disease.

As we are energetic beings, all pain and suffering is stored on the cellular level. By the time, there is a physical ailment, it means you weren't paying attention to the tiny whispers, to that inner voice earlier. Your body is sending a signal that something is not right. Be your own friend and forgive yourself, the other person and the situation you were in.

Forgiveness will open doors for you to move through and forward. It will ease your step, it will reduce your stress, and improve your overall well being. If you want to be happy, start with forgiveness.

"When a situation comes your way that is unfavorable, you always have three choices on how to respond. Eliminate it by removing yourself, change it, if you cannot change it, accept it."
– Michael Beckwith

In the stillness of meditation, we begin to see our wounds with clarity and compassion. Forgiveness doesn't mean condoning what has happened or dismissing the pain—it means releasing the hold that the pain has over us.

Guided meditations focusing on forgiveness can be particularly powerful, helping you to visualize the release of anger, resentment, and hurt. By forgiving, we free ourselves from the chains of the past and open the door to emotional freedom.

Practice forgiveness daily to relieve stress, anxiety, grudges you hold about others. If you want to have peace in your life, sustainable and long lasting, then make it a habit to forgive.

Gratitude is a natural counterpart to forgiveness. Once we have made peace with the past, we can begin to appreciate the present and all that it holds. Gratitude is more than just recognizing the good things in life—it is an active practice of acknowledging and cherishing them. Appreciating the little things in life, as they lead to big things.

In meditation, we can cultivate gratitude by focusing on the simple joys that are often overlooked: the warmth of the sun, the sound of birds singing, the comfort of a loved one's voice. By regularly practicing gratitude meditation, we train our minds to seek out and savor these moments of beauty and joy, even in the midst of hardship.

Gratitude also shifts our perspective from what we lack to what we have. This shift is transformative, especially for those recovering from trauma. It helps to rebuild a sense of abundance and sufficiency, replacing feelings of emptiness and despair with contentment and hope.

The true power of meditation lies in its ability to extend beyond the cushion or chair and into daily life. As we continue to practice forgiveness and gratitude in our meditation, these qualities begin to infuse our everyday experiences. We become more patient, more compassionate, and more resilient. We start to respond to challenges with grace rather than anger, to see opportunities where we once saw obstacles.

Daily meditation practice, even if just for a few minutes, can be a cornerstone of emotional resilience. Over time, these moments of stillness and reflection build upon one another, creating a foundation of inner peace that can weather any storm.

In the end, meditation is about movement—a gentle, steady movement toward healing, peace, and self-discovery. Through the practices of forgiveness and gratitude, we move beyond mere survival and step into a life filled with purpose and joy. The stillness we cultivate in meditation is not an absence of action, but rather a profound and powerful force for change, one that propels us toward the life we are meant to live.

So, as you close this chapter, I invite you to take a deep breath and begin. Start small, just five minutes a day, and let the ripple effects of your practice unfold. Each moment of stillness will carry you further into the clarity, peace, and strength you deserve. Meditation is not about escaping life, but about fully embracing it—one breath, one step, one day at a time. This is your moment to create lasting change; let today be the day you begin.

HOBBIES

⤨

"Always re-invent yourself. Always try new things; new food, new hobbies, meet new people. That will keep your life from becoming stagnant and boring. And you will have a lot more fun!" – Lisa Bedrick

---

*A*s we grow older we get buried with responsibilities, errands and commitments. We get inundated with never ending to do lists and mile long agendas. We become adults, we become serious, we forget our childhood dreams. We have things to do and bills to pay.

Often, we hear that hobbies are for kids, but I disagree. No matter how old or young you are, you still have a little five year old voice inside of you and you're allowed to let him or her come out and play once in a while.

Through actively pursuing your personal interest you discover who you are, you let in and explore your creative side.

Do you find yourself working all the time?

Have you created a space in your schedule for you to feed your soul?

Through hobbies I discovered a new dimension to life I didn't know existed.

It shows up as a new sparkle in my eyes, a bounce in my step, a breath of fresh air, and the groove or flow that feels aligned with what my heart desires.

I've joined Toastmasters club through my work and embarked on an extraordinary journey of public speaking. Public speaking ranks as high as the fear of death.

Joining Toastmasters allowed me to embrace and conquer my fear of public speaking. I have gained confidence and experienced the delicious energy of having an audience at your fingertips, hanging on to your every word.

Have you ever done something that felt scary on the inside but you did it anyway?

There is magic that happens on the other side of fear. It must be felt to be understood.

It can feel like a sudden burst of courage and confidence to do great things, bigger things, things you thought were impossible. Instead of thinking of the worst case scenario, you suddenly start asking, wow, what else can I do.

There is plenty of untapped potential in each one of us, it's been said and studies reveal we only use a fraction of what we are really capable of.

You don't need to feel limited by what you know, there is always room to grow and discover hidden gems while pursuing your hobbies. Armed with curiosity by your side, the sky's the limit with what you can conjure up and discover.

One of the gems I discovered was singing.

It opened a great avenue as I delved into the magical world of music. At first, it was like peeking through the covers, getting a little taste. I wasn't great at it right away but I kept exploring and trying new techniques.

One of the immediate benefits I have received from pursuing my passion to sing is the improvement of my mental health. I get to use both sides of my brain, the analytical and the creative one to unleash my imagination. I feel more present and engaged in my day to day life and my life is enriched by the experiences and people I meet through music. I hired a voice coach and took lessons twice a week during my lunch hour. Every couple of months the voice coach organized recitals and I got to meet her other students. We all sang our prepared songs and finished off by singing everyone's favorite impromptu.

I also enrolled my child to take lessons in a nearby music school. When they didn't work out, I decided to go instead. I took lessons there once per week. They also had recitals twice a year, so I was able to practice my craft and sing on stage in front of a live audience. This was such an incredible experience.

On one such occasion, I got to perform in one of the oldest rock clubs in New York City, the Bitter End rock club. To my surprise, I wasn't the only adult student in the music school for kids as there are two other locations, and so the adult band was formed. There I was, thinking that it was too late for me to start to learn because I was in the midst of kids taking lessons. When the band was formed, I discovered I was the youngest. There was a retired school teacher in his 70s who had a gig every night of the week and traveled around the country. He played bass guitar and had an active social life as if he was in his 30s. There was a dentist in his 50s playing the guitar and composing virtuoso self taught piano pieces. He started taking lessons at the school as a result of his son's interest in music. We had a stay at home mom of two teenagers who was a drummer. She was in her 40s. And then, there was me, a vocalist in my 30s. I said "I'll sing anything you want me to" as I was excited for the opportunity to be a part of the band and to perform on stage. We had rehearsals every Saturday for three months straight before the concert. When the day of the show came the club was filled to the brim with kids, their parents and friends. We were the only adult band. Our set time was pushed by a couple of hours as every band performed. Finally it was our time to be on stage. We had two songs, *Living for the City* by Stevie Wonder and *Pride and Joy* by Stevie Ray Vaughan. These weren't songs I usually sang, but they were good for the band and I was grateful for the opportunity. I wasn't a great singer back then, but the experience was absolutely incredible. I loved every bit of it. We received a standing ovation and a round of applause.

Argentine tango, much like singing, was a deep passion of mine. During my marriage, I set it aside because my spouse didn't want me dancing with other men. I explored all kinds of ballroom styles, but Argentine tango always held my heart. It offered a freedom of expression unlike any other. Every dance felt like a unique masterpiece—no two were ever the same. Once you master the basics, you can infuse your own flair, while other styles feel rigid and confined. For me, tango was even more intimate than sex; it awakened my soul and electrified me with the sensation of being fully present with my partner. In those moments, the outside world vanished—it was just me, my partner, and the music, swirling together in something so sensual, so magical. Each dance was a chance to create something beautiful and new. What I loved most was the endless creativity, tracing the floor with intricate footwork, painting a fresh canvas with every step. My soul soared as our feet crafted figure eights, pirouettes, ganchos, and boleos—an intricate masterpiece woven by two souls in love with the dance.

"To be really happy and really safe, one ought to have at least two or three hobbies, and they must all be real." – Winston Churchill

Do you have a hobby or a heart's desire to pursue something new?

When learning a skill or pursuing a hobby, set an intention to be committed 100%.

I believe life is about experiences. As you come and leave this world by yourself, you cannot take your earthly possessions, but you can take the experiences you had and that is what makes life worthwhile.

It is never too late to discover what you always wanted to learn or try. You are not too old, too busy, too young, too rich or too poor. Whatever is important, you can make time for that. We all have 24 hours in a day and a choice in how we want to spend them.

What do you want to create with the time you're alive?

There is never a perfect moment as life unfolds in the way that you allow it to. You create every moment of every day whether you like it or not. Your words, thoughts and actions dictate your human experience.

You can think of life as a play where you are the actor.

I encourage you to go ahead and pursue your hobbies, not for anyone else's sake but your own.

Who knows what you can create when you are letting it all come through you.

The most important bit to remember is that you came here to have an experience, so live your life without regret and do the things that make you happy, do not wait another moment for the perfect opportunity to arrive.

Create some space for your hobbies, revel in them and allow your creativity to come out. Make it a practice, a non-negotiable element of who you are and see how your life flourishes.

BEING PRESENT

"*Unease, anxiety, tension, stress, worry — all forms of fear — are caused by too much future, and not enough presence.*"

– *Eckhart Tolle*

---

*I*n our desire to always rush or be in a hurry we often miss life's golden moments. We forget all about being and keep doing. We are human beings and came here to have a living experience.

Why is being present so important?

Being present is essential because it allows us to fully experience and engage with life in a meaningful way. When we are truly in the moment, we connect more deeply with ourselves, others, and the world around us. It enhances our ability to focus, reduces stress, and helps us appreciate the beauty and subtleties of each experience.

Being present fosters emotional awareness, leading to better relationships and decision-making, as we respond with clarity rather than being distracted or overwhelmed. Ultimately, it prevents life from passing us by, allowing us to live with intention, joy, and fulfillment.

Life moves quickly, especially with rapid technological advancements, and our minds struggle to keep up. To truly experience life, we must slow down, quiet the external noise, and reconnect with ourselves. Life is a collection of moments, and if we're constantly rushing, we may reach the end feeling like we never truly lived—just following others' expectations.

Many people sleepwalk through life, only realizing too late that they weren't really living. Don't let that happen to you. In this fast-paced world, being present is essential and must be consciously practiced to live fully.

We do this more naturally when we are little kids, feeling like there is no moment like the present.

Have you ever noticed that when you are around kids?

They are so focused on what is happening right in front of them, they aren't thinking about what could have been, all their essence is in the present moment. There is magic to that.

When something unpleasant happens, a child may feel like it will last forever and have a big emotional reaction. Similarly, if you tell them something exciting will happen in a week, they get excited right away and will constantly ask, "Is it time yet?" every chance they get.

So, we knew all this when we were young, but overtime, the pressures of conforming to societal norms pushed it aside.

What once came naturally to us now feels lost, but the beauty is, we can choose to remember it and bring it back into our daily lives. In today's culture, where multitasking reigns supreme, we often end up distracted more than anything else. Juggling too many things at once pulls us in different directions, leaving us only half-present in any given moment. As we rush from task to task, we risk letting life slip by, feeling as though we've achieved little despite our constant activity. The more we divide our attention, the more we miss out on the richness of being fully engaged in the here and now.

Being present came really handy and I truly believe it played a crucial role in getting me through my recent visit to Sedona, Arizona. Sedona is a magical place that offers breathtaking beauty of the magnificent rock formations, open vistas and grandeur of mother nature. My daily hiking opportunities to visit the vortexes required some climbing. I am not an avid rock climber, not by far but with the help of our awesome guide it was possible. However, it required me to really be present. It was painstakingly clear that if I don't pay attention to every single step that I take, I not only sabotage myself but also could cause harm to others that are following in my steps.

There were people above and people below so it was important that everyone keep a consistent rhythm. Being extra careful how and where I placed my feet and how I balanced my body, I made it to the top of the Cathedral Rock. This was a sunrise hike and glorious Sedona offered its beautiful vistas every step of the way. The journey up was totally worth the view that was waiting for me at the top. Oftentimes we get discouraged when our goal is so far out of reach, we might question why we are even in pursuit of it. Focusing your attention on every step of the way and then celebrating that small victory will reinforce your belief and prove to your mind why you started.

Attention is the biggest commodity you have in the game of life. Where attention goes, energy flows. Ever wonder why when you are doing something you enjoy, time just flies. You are fully there, engaged, feeling, breathing, sensing every moment. You are experiencing the state of flow. That is what many artists, singers, writers and other creators experience when they are perfecting their craft.

"If you want to conquer the anxiety of life, live in the moment, live in the breath." – Amit Ray

There are many who want to hijack your attention. TV, news, advertisements, social media and so on. You must be the guardian that discerns where the attention is spent and what is allowed in your environment. That can only happen when you are aware of how and where you place your attention.

In every situation and experience it is 20% of what happens and 80% how you react to it. Too often, something only lasted a fraction of a time can have a devastating effect on the rest of your life, because you linger on too much on who said what and how you felt; sending yourself back in the past, reliving past traumas only activates the same parts of your brain and sends you further back. Instead of seeking relief and creating a better future, you keep recreating the past. You are missing out on the present and not working towards your future.

The future is created in the present moment.

The thoughts you think about become your reality, just like the radio station that broadcasts a signal to attract a certain kind of listener who likes what they hear. Your thinking broadcasts the frequency of your desire and what you think about, you attract.

When you are being present you place deliberate attention to the thoughts you are thinking that bring about the outcome, people, places and experiences into your orbit.

It is important to pay close attention to what you think about and become the observer of your experience. In the beginning it may feel difficult to do so, but with practice it becomes second nature.

Just like the scientist who performs experiments and studies the outcome, allow yourself to experiment, especially that you have nothing to lose and everything to gain.

Practice placing deliberate attention on your thoughts and see what happens.

Recipe for Being Present

Next time you are outside, remove all distractions and really take in the nature with all your senses: tune in to the sounds of the birds, or the bubbling of a brook, feel the cool breeze against your skin, see the marvelous colors of an autumn sky, taste that tantalizing morsel of food, smell the morning's crisp air, stretch your body and absorb all that. Focus your attention by aligning your thoughts with the full experience of your senses.

You are being present.

When you hug somebody, be fully there. Let go of your to do lists and errands, and in that brief moment, immerse yourself in the connection. Feel the warmth, notice how your shoulders relax, and sense the tension melting away. In that space, you'll discover that you are safe, protected and loved.

Being present doesn't always require grand gestures, it can be as simple as setting a daily reminder on your phone with a word or phrase that resonates. Those could be messages to self, full sentences or simple words. When the reminder goes off, pause.

Reflect on its meaning, feel it deeply, and ask yourself how you can embody it today.

What does it mean to you?

How does it make you feel?

How can you practice this today?

This doesn't have to be long, only a minute of your time to train yourself to focus on the present moment. As with any habit, repetition is key, the more you practice, the better you will become.

Continue to explore your own moments when you feel present. Maybe you are singing, composing poetry, speaking in front of an audience, or painting.

When you immerse yourself in something you love, time fades, distractions fall away, and you become fully alive in the moment. That's the magic of being present—where true joy and connection are found.

Where can you be more present in your life?

BECOMING FREE FROM VICTIMHOOD

$\mathcal{CSP}$

"The victim mindset dilutes the human potential. By not accepting personal responsibility for our circumstances, we greatly reduce our power to change them." – Steve Maraboli

---

*V*ictimhood is when someone feels stuck in a mindset where they believe bad things always happen to them, and they have no control over the situation. It can make you feel powerless, like life is unfair and everything is out of your hands. When you're in this mindset, it is easy to blame others or circumstances for your problems, instead of taking responsibility for your choices. This can keep you from growing or changing things for the better, leaving you feeling frustrated and trapped. Learning to break free from victimhood means recognizing your own power to shape your life, even when things get tough.

Every event and experience in our life came about as a result of our thoughts, words and actions. Thanks to delayed manifestation, you see the results of your thinking a bit down the line. If materialization was instantaneous, we would have placed more careful attention to what we think about and what we utter into existence every second of every day. We have tremendous power of choice. It is up to us to where we place our attention and deliberately create things into being.

Our time here is limited, yet we continue to poison ourselves with negative thinking, carrying grudges for years on end. We have a mountain heap of expectations and when they are unfulfilled, we fall into a pit of despair and loathing. We continuously keep the toxic past alive even though we cannot change it and continue to miss out on the present from where our future can be created. We continue living in a distorted reality of the upset mind and continue to recreate the same scenario over and over again, digging a deeper hole which would be difficult to climb out of.

All of this is not to negate the fact of mistreatment, but to let the past stay in the past and create a better future for yourself. When you are in the thick of a situation, it is tough to see or feel any different other than a victim.

Recreating negative situations is unhealthy and detrimental to our physical health as well. Our bodies are energetic impulses and emotions are currents carrying signals alerting the system if something is out of whack or if something is in bliss. They don't go anywhere; they are just circulating throughout the system carrying messages to the mailbox of our mind. When the mailbox gets full, it starts overflowing with all of those negative events, thoughts and ideas and penetrates the healthy system by turning on itself. Prolonged inattention may manifest in a disease. The gravity of the disease is inherent to the user and how alert they are to receiving the messages and not taking any action to counter the effect. Every time you recall toxic thoughts, parts of conversations, phrases thrown in a heat of passion, you also recall the feelings and emotions associated with those thoughts. You make all of that come alive and experience every feeling, every upset, every pain and hurt all over again. Your mind cannot tell if something is past, present or future, imaginary or fake, truth or lie, it takes everything as is, literally. You are the one conducting the orchestra of your mind. The same parts of the brain light up when you think about a past or a future event. For the mind everything is happening right here right now. Everything is a present moment reality.

Sometimes you may feel like a masochist constantly spinning the picture that is upsetting, and making yourself sick in the process. You may create stories that are distorted or taken out of context and allow them to lead your life. The unprocessed emotions of the past are evoked and layer after layer added one on top of the other, accumulated over time, and as I mentioned earlier, these emotions may manifest in a disease.

Are you making yourself sick with your own unhealthy thoughts?

"Stop validating your victim mentality. Shake off your self-defeating drama and embrace your innate ability to recover and achieve."

– Steve Maraboli

The more you focus on the problem, on what is not working, on what is broken, on what feels unjust or what is debilitating and hopeless the bigger it becomes. It feels like a room with no way out. Remember, nothing can change for the better by constantly regurgitating the intrusive thoughts of the past. The mind that created the problem must change in order to arrive at the solution. As I remember, the definition of insanity is doing the same thing and expecting a different result.

Good news, solutions do exist!

Think of the problem as a gift, it can teach you a lesson, a positive lesson you can walk away with so that you make a better decision next time.

The impact of staying in victimhood for me was huge. It not only affected me, but my relationships, career and mental health were also shaken. As you wouldn't expect a lemon to produce orange juice, you cannot expect a bright personality from someone who is in a state of victimhood. All the toxicity is spilled over into the relationships as well, you develop a temperament, which later becomes a part of your personality. You are then associated and thought about like that negative person, who constantly complains about their life, blaming others and not taking any action in the direction of change.

Little things may trigger you into oblivion. A mountain of expectations of how life is supposed to be and why it is not working in your specific situation. Your mental health suffers as a result. You may have thoughts of unworthiness, your outlook on life diminishes, everything feels gray, and life feels as if it has no meaning.

You are missing out on the present and the beautiful future you can create for yourself. I have no vivid recollection of when my son took his first steps and uttered his first words. I was physically there but those events aren't stitched up in my memory like they were when my daughter was born. My outer shell was there, performing duties and obligations that were expected of me, but my inner core was missing. My mind was clouded by the unfairness of the situation, by how I am supposed to go on living, figuring things out on my own, being a mom and a dad and still asking why did this happen to me? What did I do to deserve this? I thought I was being punished for being a good wife and mom. I never argued or raised my voice, always agreeing and going along, being complacent of keeping peace, sweeping things under the rug. Meanwhile I didn't feel that I had enough experience to do my best job of being a parent. I was still learning, and I don't believe I will ever stop.

Being a victim can feel easy, giving up responsibility and making yourself believe that somehow it's someone else's fault that your life turned out the way it did. They were making all these decisions and you were simply following along. We all have freedom to choose. We have the ability to decide what we consider the truth. My truth is true for me but you could have a totally different kind of truth. Each person's beliefs manifest and resonate to the outside world what you believe to be true. Your mind will always confirm to you, it will seek examples to prove you right. It does not know any different and can only conjure up what you create, your thoughts and ideas of how life should be. Your thoughts influence the world around you. The world is a mirror reflecting back to you, your inner state. You can fight about it, be enraged about it, yet it can't show you anything different other than what you believe and expect out of life.

Victimhood found me after my breakup and suddenly I became a single parent of two very young kids. I thought at the time that I had wasted the best years of my life with the wrong person. I was devastated and didn't know how I was going to continue living. I blamed everything on my life's circumstances, and it wasn't until I took responsibility for my life that I was able to realize that it was the choices that I made that led me to the life I had created.

It is a tough decision, taking responsibility, whereas all your life you have listened to other figures of authority. Being told what to eat, what to wear, how to behave and how to think. We build trust in these figures of authority, we trust doctors with our health and therapists with our mental health, yet we forget to trust and listen to ourselves. We somehow think that trusting others will solve all of our problems, but maybe it is our unwillingness to take responsibility for our own actions. Of course that responsibility means there is no one to blame if we fail. Becoming an observer of my life instead of blindly following along and being swept up by the strong current was the answer. Every event is here to teach a lesson. Unfortunately, over time small little things accumulate into a snowball that doesn't fit under the rug anymore. Small tiny things drive people apart, they become a wedge in the relationship which drives them away. People come together in a relationship from different backgrounds and upbringings, and it is understandable that each one carries a set of values and beliefs that are true for them. Yet some beliefs, especially if they are a core part of your personality, must not be crossed.

Compromises are possible if both agree and speak about that and make it known to the other person. Contrary to popular belief we cannot read each other's mind and therefore must speak up and establish a level of communication that is necessary for the relationship to survive. Often, we have all that in a job setting, yet when it comes to personal relationships that aspect is missing.

There are detrimental long term effects that can transpire the longer you continue to stay in the victim state. Trapped emotions layered one on top of the other without any release mechanism will create a disease over time. Not to mention staying in the victim state does not solve anything, it just creates a bigger hole and makes it harder and longer to climb out of. Somehow, we humans like to make our life difficult when it does not have to be. If we only knew that the power of the words we speak and thoughts we think bring about the reality we live in. Unfortunately, our ego wants to feel validated and reminds us how wounded we are.

The road to recovery begins with the acknowledgement that current reality no longer serves your highest good. You are tired of the life you are living and something must change.

Until you reach that breaking point, no matter what anyone says will stray you away.

Standing on a platform, feeling tired of the mad rush of each morning, the never-ending feeling of not really living but simply existing took a toll. That was the moment I decided to make a change. I did not have the tools at the time, but deep down I knew, there must be more to this thing called life. I wanted to wake up happy and be content throughout the day, living life according to my design, being and doing things that bring me joy.

Are you ready to take responsibility for your life?

This is an important step in reclamation and owning all your actions and choices. You no longer have others to blame, you must find a way out. Your thinking got you into the rut, now it is time to dig yourself out.

Are you ready to learn from your mistakes? Are you looking for solutions?

Growth Mindset

This is a belief that abilities and intelligence can be developed through dedication and hard work. In contrast a fixed mindset sees abilities as innate and unchangeable. Growth mindset allows flexibility in thinking, you are no longer scared of change, you are looking for solutions. One example that comes to mind from my life, when the mailbox broke and needed fixing, I looked for ways to do so. The challenge was drilling through brick and I didn't have any prior experience in that arena. I did drill holes in drywall, but this material was new to me. As I found out a special drill bit was needed for that, so I proceeded to perform the task until it was complete. Another time, an oven door fell, and after watching several YouTube videos, took up that challenge and fixed the door.

In a work setting, it is about seeking solutions and finding the people who can answer your query and not resting until you do. In a relationship, you might find that it is not about winning an argument but coming to an agreement with each other, it is about not being stuck that something can only be done one way. Something as simple as how one partner fills up the dishwasher and another does it in a different way.

Thoughts, situations and beliefs that we have can lead to us being triggered. All of these get developed during our formative years. It is the environment where we grew up, what we've seen and heard from our parents, caregivers, school teachers, and bosses. Then our own experience plays a role as well as they intertwine and reinforce the ideas we had when growing up. We add "salt to the wound" that fixates our ability and encourages our understanding of how things are. If something was done one way for decades on end, sometimes it is impossible to see it any other way. We willingly accept the limitations of our mind if our past shows evidence of lackluster results, failures and unacceptance of any kind.

The psychological mechanisms such as fear of failure, avoidance of challenges and the desire for validation add an additional protective layer that prevents from breaking out of the fixed mindset. Fear of failure can have you trapped from even starting the thing. Especially if in the past you've already experienced failures, it may be difficult to expect anything more. You don't want to disillusion yourself and miss out on the chance of what can happen. In reality, there is no failure, it seemingly does not exist. You only fail if you stop trying. Every failure acts as feedback on what not to do next time. Remember when you were little, you didn't stop trying after your first unsuccessful attempt to stand up or take a first step. You fell and got up and tried again. You were not afraid of what anyone said or thought, and you didn't contemplate thousands of ways that you could fail. You kept going until you succeeded and were able to hold your balance and take your first steps. You weren't conditioned yet by society of who you must be and how you must act. You simply believed; you were curious about the possibility of what you might discover. Your senses were sharpened, everything looked interesting to explore.

Avoidance of challenges might show up as you no longer want to put yourself in situations that would break you out of your comfort zone. You fear that you may not possess the necessary skills or intelligence to successfully complete the challenging task/project/conversation. You worry about making mistakes or not meeting expectations, which could damage your self-esteem and reputation. Due to these fixed mindset beliefs, you prefer to stay within your comfort zone, where you feel competent and confident.

You perceive the challenge as a threat to your sense of security and familiarity, preferring to avoid it rather than risk failure or embarrassment. You convince yourself that the challenge is too difficult or beyond your capabilities, rationalizing that you are better suited for tasks that align with your existing skills and expertise. You avoid investing time and effort into learning new skills or seeking assistance, believing that success should come naturally without exerting extra effort. When faced with setbacks or obstacles, you quickly become discouraged and unmotivated. You interpret challenges as evidence of your incompetence or inadequacy, reinforcing fixed mindset beliefs about your limitations and reinforcing your reluctance to take on future challenges.

Desire for validation can also reinforce fixed mindset beliefs. If you've always been praised for your natural intelligence and quick understanding of concepts in school, overtime you begin to internalize the belief that your worth is tied to your academic achievements and innate abilities. You become increasingly focused on seeking validation from others, striving to maintain your image as the "smart" person who excels effortlessly. As a result, you develop a fixed mindset towards learning and challenges. You avoid tasks or subjects that you perceive as difficult or where you might struggle, fearing that failure would tarnish your reputation and undermine your sense of self-worth. You become reluctant to ask for help or seek feedback, as you believe that doing so would reveal your limitations and diminish other's perceptions of your intelligence.

Freedom from victimhood begins with reclaiming your narrative. Acknowledge your past experiences but refuse to let them define your future. Shift from "Why did this happen to me?" to "What can I learn from this?" Recognize your power to shape your own story, choosing to see yourself as a survivor and thriver, not a victim. Embrace responsibility for your emotions and reactions, knowing that true empowerment lies in your response, not in the events themselves. Through this perspective shift, you reclaim control over your life, transforming pain into strength and adversity into opportunity for growth.

But continuously, with training and redirecting of your mind this could be a tool with which to navigate life. Viewing each situation as an observer and studying life like the scientist who performs an experiment, revealing not so obvious parts. Studying the event and looking for positive lessons in a negative experience. These could be the "hard pill" to swallow or an ugly truth that you get to learn about yourself. Yet the lessons are what we must extract and move forward with the newly obtained knowledge into the future. Making better decisions with each next experience.

DEALING WITH OVERWHELM

❦

"Accept responsibility for your life. You know that it is you who will get you where you want to go, no one else." – Les Brown

---

Overwhelm can impact all areas of life. Let's define overwhelm: it is a state of being emotionally, mentally, or physically overloaded often characterized by feelings of stress, anxiety, or confusion, to the point where it becomes challenging to cope effectively. Overwhelm isn't just a passing feeling; it can have profound effects on mental health. Left unchecked, it can exacerbate symptoms of anxiety, depression, and post-traumatic stress disorder (PTSD). It can disrupt daily life in significant ways. It may impair concentration, memory, and decision-making abilities, making it difficult to perform tasks at work or school. Additionally, it can strain relationships and hinder social interactions, further isolating you when you already feel lost and misunderstood.

The toll of overwhelm isn't limited to mental health, it can also manifest physically. Chronic stress, which often accompanies overwhelm, can weaken the immune system, increase the risk of heart problems, and contribute to other health issues. So, addressing overwhelm is crucial for safeguarding overall wellbeing.

Let's look at what happens from a scientific point of view. Overwhelm triggers the body's stress response system, also known as the "flight-or-fight" response which activates the sympathetic nervous system and releases stress hormones like cortisol and adrenaline. This is a great response mechanism as it is the one responsible for keeping you safe. When you're crossing the street and suddenly a car appears out of nowhere, it is this response that jerks you back and keeps you alive. The timing of this response was designed to last a few seconds, unfortunately what happens in the modern world is this same response lasts for hours, days, months and years. This prolonged exposure to cortisol and adrenaline can affect the brain's structure and function, particularly the amygdala, responsible for processing emotions and the prefrontal cortex, involved in decision-making and problem-solving.

Suddenly minor things cause more havoc than intended. All emotions want is to be felt and then let go, not hold on to them for dear life. Chronic stress can disrupt the balance of neurotransmitters such as serotonin, dopamine, and norepinephrine, contributing to symptoms of anxiety, depression and mood disturbances.

"None of us can go back and start a new beginning, but all of us can start a new day and make a new ending."

– Lisa Lieberman-Wang

These are the many ways of how overwhelm can manifest including, intrusive thoughts, emotional volatility, physical tension, and difficulty focusing or making decisions. Intrusive thoughts are unwelcome, involuntary thoughts, images, or ideas that can be distressing and difficult to control. These show up as recurring worries, fears, or memories related to the traumatic event. This leads to heightened anxiety, rumination, and feelings of helplessness. You can experience intrusive thoughts as flashbacks to the traumatic event, vivid memories, or catastrophic scenarios about the future. Coping may require strategies such as mindfulness techniques, grounding exercises, and cognitive-behavioral therapy to challenge negative thought patterns and promote emotional regulation.

Overwhelm doesn't happen overnight, as it is a daily neglect on the part of us listening to our own body. Oftentimes you take care of others and forget to take care of yourself. Understandably so, as you try to hold your ship afloat and put out fires as they arise, little by little even if for your own detriment. You were not meant to hold it all together, you are in your human experience, discovering and unfolding in every way. If you are by yourself holding down the fort, then take it easy on you and pay attention when your body is signaling you to slow down and take rest if necessary.

Overwhelm at work

Stress factors such as heavy workloads, tight deadlines and job insecurity can lead to feelings of exhaustion, burnout, and disengagement. Little by little these things can creep up on you. I've experienced this myself many times over the years. At first it is manageable and then it spikes out of control. It all goes back to maintaining the daily rituals, when those things slide, it is like the foundation that is being washed away and then there is nothing to hold on to. All you want is to go to sleep and not wake up anymore. When the resources are drained it is only up to you to restore them. The unfortunate part is that it is difficult for others to see what you are going through. They might notice your curt remarks but wouldn't understand where those came from. This is an internal battle that many fight on their own.

When dealing with job insecurity, it is tough especially when the sense of security was ingrained into our upbringing. While it is ephemeral as companies have that clause of at will employment. Technically speaking they can get rid of you anytime they choose, just as you can walk away from a job that isn't suitable. Yet we yearn for that sense of stability and security which comes from the lack mindset.

In an attempt to cope with overwhelm, we sometimes turn to unhealthy behaviors such as substance abuse, self-harm, or avoidance. These coping mechanisms provide temporary relief but ultimately exacerbate the underlying issues. By addressing overwhelm directly, you can avoid falling into destructive patterns and cultivate healthier coping strategies.

Traumatic experiences can leave deep emotional wounds that require attention and care to heal. So, you can create space for processing emotions, confronting unresolved trauma, and embarking on a journey of recovery. This is essential for reclaiming a sense of agency, autonomy, and empowerment in your life.

Overwhelm showed up in my life the moment I was faced with having to figure everything out by myself. After you've been living with someone for close to a decade you may have eased your grasp on things, be it managing finances, taking care of repairs, getting a car or a loan, being a mom and dad to your kids and wearing many other hats at the same time as well. As you try to make sure nothing falls apart, you find yourself as a joggler having 25 balls in the air all at the same time and God forbid if one of them falls. Do it all with a smile on your face, keep it together because the world is watching.

When I became a single parent nine years ago, I was the outlier, as everyone around me was happily married. Nowadays, there are single parents everywhere, somehow it is the new norm. The world of today is fast-paced and interconnected, yet we are more disconnected from ourselves. I was overwhelmed with emotions of helplessness, intrusive thoughts were mine companions, often suggesting what I should've said, done, or been different. After all, I was in uncharted territory, somewhere I've never been before. Why I was expecting certainty or knowledge at that point is beyond my understanding. Yet, being raised as always holding your shit together, you continue to keep holding the shit, even when it is time to let it go. You don't have to carry everything on your own, you are allowed to make mistakes and you're also allowed to ask for help. Asking for help wasn't my strong suit since I was always on the other side of giving help to others, but not on the receiving end.

"It is during our darkest moments that we must focus to see the light."

– Aristotle Onassis

So how does one get back on the road of reclamation and getting your power back?

By addressing overwhelm and learning effective coping strategies, you can strengthen your resilience and enhance capacity to navigate future challenges. This resilience serves as a protective factor against the negative effects of trauma and overwhelm. While those can be deeply painful experiences, they also represent learning opportunities for growth and transformation. By addressing overwhelm head on, you can harness the lessons learned from your experiences, cultivate self-awareness and insight, and emerge from adversity with newfound strength, wisdom, and resilience.

Some of the coping mechanisms and practices to deal with overwhelm include prioritization and time management, stress reduction techniques, setting boundaries and saying no.

• Having a schedule or a routine can prove beneficial at addressing overwhelm. Yes routine doesn't sound all that exciting, however in the routine you can find freedom. Finding what works for you is key.

• Some people utilize the power of making lists and crossing things off. If you have a very long list, do not attempt to solve everything at once but prioritize your top three main tasks for the day. Checking in at the end of the day to evaluate yourself on the job well done or whether there is room for improvement. After all we only improve what we measure, what we pay attention to.

• When it comes to time management, time blocking could be beneficial. First you need to understand where you spend your time and then color code accordingly what needs to be done and at what time. If you are great at something, do that thing and outsource something you are not great at, so that you can focus and spend your time and energy effectively.

Stress reduction techniques include changing your state, unburdening your schedule and creating more space in your life.

• Changing your state is as easy as switching your activities, if let's say you've been sitting for too long in front of a screen, getting up and stretching, or dancing, or getting a glass of water would engage your other muscle groups and would change your state. Exposing yourself to a nature walk can do wonders for your mental health. Just the other day, I really felt depleted and disengaged, so taking myself on the beach, transporting my scenery and surroundings really improved my mood. Another powerful technique for stress reduction is reframing negative thought patterns.

• Sometimes we overwork our brain to the point of exhaustion by constant worrying, and engaging into unhelpful thought processes. One way to reframe your thoughts is to give yourself a gentle flinch of a rubber band to remind yourself you're exhibiting destructive behaviors.

• Having a mantra to speak over your thoughts is another great tool to practice.

In moments of overwhelm, it's easy to feel lost in the chaos of endless demands and responsibilities. However, by recognizing our triggers, implementing practical tools for organizing our thoughts and tasks, and fostering mental resilience, we can transform that chaos into clarity. Overcoming overwhelm isn't about eliminating challenges but about equipping ourselves with the strategies to face them head-on, one step at a time. Remember, it's not about perfection but progress—each small, focused action brings us closer to a life of calm, balance, and fulfillment.

ENVIRONMENT

"Surround yourself with what you love, whether it's family, pets, keepsakes, music, plants, hobbies, whatever." – George Carlin

In our quest to reclaim our lives, we often focus on our inner strengths and choices. But what if I told you that the environment around you, the people who surround you, are the silent architects molding the foundation of your life?

This chapter will explore the unexpected truths about how your environment plays a pivotal role in your journey of self-reclamation.

We often hear the phrase, "You are what you eat," emphasizing the importance of a healthy diet for our physical well-being. But this concept extends far beyond food; it encompasses everything we consume—what we see, feel, experience, and the people we surround ourselves with. Our environment shapes us in ways we often overlook, influencing our thoughts, emotions, and ultimately, our identity.

Imagine a cucumber placed in a jar of pickles. No matter how fresh and distinct it starts out, it eventually absorbs the flavors around it, transforming into a pickle itself. This analogy illustrates a powerful truth: just like the cucumber, we are deeply affected by the environments we immerse ourselves in. The people we interact with, the media we consume, the places we frequent—all of these external stimuli seep into our subconscious, shaping our thoughts, behaviors, and attitudes.

Our brains are wired to adapt and respond to the stimuli around us. We absorb the emotions, beliefs, and energies of those we spend time with, often without even realizing it. This is because humans are social creatures, designed to mirror and learn from each other. While this ability has its benefits—such as fostering empathy and learning new skills—it also means that we are vulnerable to absorbing negativity, fear, and limiting beliefs from our surroundings.

Consider how many of your daily thoughts are recycled from the previous day. Research shows that 95% of the thoughts we think today are the same as yesterday, and for many, these thoughts are filled with self-doubt, anxiety, and negativity. This mental repetition is akin to soaking in a jar of "pickle water," where the continuous exposure to negative stimuli—

whether it's toxic relationships, fear-driven media, or a stressful work environment—slowly turns our mindset sour.

As creatures of habit, we tend to stick with familiar thought patterns, even when they no longer serve us. If the environment we are in constantly feeds us negative or limiting beliefs, these ideas can begin to feel like our own. Over time, we internalize them, and they become part of our identity, influencing how we see ourselves and the world around us.

Imagine waking up each day and immediately being bombarded with stress—perhaps from the news, social media, or a difficult family dynamic. These negative inputs can set the tone for your entire day, making it harder to break free from a cycle of worry, fear, and self-sabotage. Just as the cucumber cannot resist turning into a pickle when submerged in pickle brine, it's difficult for us to resist the impact of a toxic environment.

Have you ever felt like you were soaking in a toxic environment?

I didn't have an uplifting environment in my life, and I didn't want to turn into a pickle, so I went after the light in other places. I felt lost and in my quest to find who I was, I first pursued my passions and then found people who share common interests. I found positive environments for each area of my life: singing, dancing, painting and personal development.

"Your environment influences your mindset." — *Robin S. Sharma*

So, what is the answer to this dilemma, how do you dig your-self out of the uncooperative surroundings, how do you pluck yourself out and make the change?

Just as cucumber can be placed in different liquids to change its flavor, we have the power to alter our surroundings and, in turn, our internal landscape. By consciously choosing uplifting, positive influences, we can transform our "jar" into an environment that fosters growth, happiness, and resilience.

Firstly, it is important to recognize what is occurring, some-times we don't even see what is happening until it is too late. Acknowledgement is the first step. When you want to change and everything is pulling against you remind yourself daily of who you are. That is where affirmations can come in handy. The daily declaration of who you are or who you want to become would serve as a reminder.

Create a vision of who you are by drafting it on a piece of paper. Do not limit yourself to any obstacles, write from the perspective of here and now, as if you already possess it. For our mind the future and past do not exist, everything is right now. When you have that list ready, make sure to recite it daily to yourself. Mornings and evenings are best, as soon as you roll out of bed and immediately before you go to sleep are the most effective times of day for this process. As we switch off our state from beta to alpha thereby bypassing critical faculty of the conscious mind imprinting the thoughts and ideas which are important. This little act of creating who you are becoming could do wonders on your overall human experience.

You can change, do not let anybody tell you otherwise. Remind yourself why and do the process. By placing deliberate focus on this task, you are sending a signal to your brain that what you are doing is important. Being open to possibilities that come your way then is the next step. As my good friend often says, be open to everything and attached to nothing, that is what being open is all about. Not having a fixed idea about something but being willing and ready to accept anything that is possible. Allow yourself to be curious and remember that it was a natural part of who you were when you were young. After all, we never stop learning, and having a beginner mindset can teach you a thing or two about life.

In the pursuit of creating who you are, seeking spaces that would promote the new you would seem beneficial. It does not just take a village to raise a child, it also takes a village to create a change, whether positive or negative you decide. People around you can significantly impact your energy levels and emotional wellbeing. Choosing positive and supportive individuals can uplift and inspire you, while toxic and negative influences can drain your vitality and hinder your progress.

So, surrounding yourself with people who embody the qualities and values you aspire to cultivate mirrors those traits within yourself, fostering personal growth and development.

Choose to spend time with people who uplift and inspire you. Seek out mentors, friends, and communities that encourage your growth and well-being. Their positive energy will help you cultivate a more optimistic mindset. I discovered these communities through different passions that I have. For each part of my life there is an outlet, there is a resource, or there is an environment that brings me closer to who I am.

Through discovering your passions, you can find a supportive environment as well. If there is something you want to pursue, go and do that, don't wait another minute! Let the parts of you reach their ultimate state, allow yourself to explore and be open to what could be possible.

BE HAPPY NOW

"One day you will wake up and there won't be any more time to do the things you've always wanted. Do it now." — Paulo Coelho

*H*appiness exists in the here and now. At any moment, with the power of our free will, we make choices and decisions about our state of being and how we want to feel, nobody is forced to feel a certain way. It is very easy to blame others that they're not fulfilling your expectations that disturb your peaceful, cheery nature. Living with expectations that you place on others is difficult, especially that you cannot control how they'll behave. The only thing you can control is your thoughts and ideas about events, people, and experiences that take place.

Did you know that it takes the same amount of energy to be miserable, angry, or sad just as it takes to be happy, joyous and excited?

All it takes is a state of mind that you can experience any time. Happiness is not found outside of you, in the next car, partner, job or business deal. It is always with you ripe for the taking. It is not unicorns and rainbows but it is moment by moment living. Sometimes it could be seeing a smile on your child's face or doing something you love or like seeing a sunrise or finding your car keys.

I am forever fascinated by the simple act of a day being born. The way the sky changes colors from crimson and scarlet to pink and beige. As I take in this beauty and vastness of the sky inadvertently a smile sneaks up onto my face.

Have you ever lost something? Remember the excitement you felt once what you lost was found? How weird it is that we remember the loss so vividly but when it was found the feeling is fleeting. It does not even register, we just carry on with our day?

Sometimes one "bad" thing piles up on top of the other and you might really find yourself in the dumps. You were already running late to an important event and now the keys are lost. They're nowhere in sight, then you find them and start driving and suddenly there is traffic everywhere preventing you from moving forward.

How do you find joy in that?

Remember that every cloud has a silver lining. Maybe the reason there is traffic is to prevent you from getting into an accident. You can turn to gratitude when you find yourself in a pickle. Think about the things that are working in your favor, instead of getting upset and giving your joy away.

Who do you allow to steal your joy?

A rude passerby on the train, a disgruntled coworker, a demanding boss or a whiny kid? Everyone has their drama and the role they like to play. You have a choice not to participate in their circus. Let their words wash over you instead of entering your safe harbor.

I remember another moment like it was yesterday. The days turned to weeks, months and years. The constant rush of daily morning commute, always running no matter what the weather or day of week. One fateful morning, after completing kids' drop off at two separate locations and looking for parking a bit longer than usual, I missed my train by mere seconds. My heart pounding loudly from all the racing and shortness of breath, I arrived at the platform all too late. The constant rush of each morning piled up and I burst into tears. These questions started coming, what is the point of all this, why am I always running yet not feeling like I am living. Each day I felt like I was getting closer to my death while not really living. Feeling like a soldier who fights in a war that never ends. There is no golden pot at the end of that rainbow.

At that moment I no longer wanted to live like that anymore, I decided to be happy again. I didn't know what or how it would be, but I simply made the decision that I needed to change. I no longer wished for the circumstances in my life to affect how I feel. I wanted to be energetic, enthusiastic, and excited to live. I wanted to be different from who I was, I wanted to be happy.

Funny story: when my son was nine years old, he completed a school project for Mother's day and to the question "what is your mom best at?" he wrote "being happy". That's the best compliment I could wish for. I couldn't believe my eyes when I read it, I had to go back and read it again and again. My child saw something in me that I didn't know I possessed.

Are people seeing happiness in you?

Are you present enough to notice?

"The present moment is filled with joy and happiness. If you are attentive, you will see it." — Thich Nhat Hanh

Sometimes happiness is found in the passion you pursue not from the pursuit but through the process of discovery of what sets your soul on fire. Finding happiness in small intangible things. Happiness is a state that you create irrespective of whether certain people are in your life. It is a state of appreciation, a state of bliss, a state of being present in your life that allows you to notice all the little moments which are strung together and create memories.

Do you have a string of memories that make you happy?

For years I was searching for that elusive state. The program of living that dictates what happiness is that you study and get good grades, then you go to college and study some more and then you build a career and start a family. You work all your life and hope that when you retire you can do something you love. All of your life is wasted on fulfilling someone else's dream.

For the longest time I was seeking happiness on the outside of me, in the new relationship, a new job opportunity, a new adventure, a new home. Always seeking this external piece as if something was missing. We always have all the resources that we need at any given time. When we place our attention on seeking external validation or external stimuli to justify happiness, we often fail to find what we seek. We have a lot of expectations about how life is supposed to be. We live with those expectations and any time they're not met, we find ourselves frustrated, anxious, angry, depressed, not our best selves.

Here is what happiness means to me. I define it as being present, so that you can witness all of life's presents without any hurry, taking your time to enjoy the experience. Let all that you do be done in love, whether making a meal or creating an artistic masterpiece, composing a song or writing a book. I believe you can design your own happiness by aligning your thoughts, words and actions. Doing what sets your soul on fire, being who you choose to be, always remembering what you give, comes back to you. Happiness for me is witnessing a sunrise, pursuing my passions of singing, painting, baking, creating new things, traveling the world, experiencing life with all of my senses, sharing what I've learned to enhance and uplift humanity, and supporting others to heal their mind, body and soul. Sharing my story and learning the stories of others who have reclaimed their life. You can find happiness in seeing the smile on your child's face, seeing a rainbow in the sky, achieving something you thought you couldn't. It can be found in the pursuit of your dream, when you wake up each morning feeling really good about who you are being!

I have a dream of singing on stage in front of a thousand people. I realize that it is not going to happen overnight. So I broke my dream into pieces, down to what it looks like on a daily basis. I practice singing, 10 minutes or more each day. Singing is also medicine for the soul, it allows me to explore how I feel, releases endorphins into my bloodstream and builds up my confidence.

Have you ever defined what happiness means to you?

What does it look like, feel like and sound like?

What does your perfect day look like?

Be sure to focus on what you do want instead of what you are trying to avoid.

This is your invitation to define happiness for yourself. Write it out without objections or limitations. Define what it means to you right here, right now, not in a distant future. Then bring these elements into your daily practices and experiences. Create a recipe that makes you happy. It doesn't have to be an elaborate plan, you could break it down into small steps and do one step at a time. Like I did above. You already have all the resources and all the tools in your possession to make yourself happy.

Wake up and follow your dreams now. Don't wait another second. Life is fleeting, before you realize it, life may be over. Appreciate it to the fullest.

SERVING OTHERS AND THE LAW OF ATTRACTION

"The best way to find yourself is to lose yourself in the service of others." – Mahatma Gandhi

*L*et's dive into the transformative power of service and how it intertwines with the Law of Attraction to create a life filled with abundance, joy and purpose. When we shift our focus from solely seeking personal gain to genuinely serving others, we tap into a higher frequency of energy that aligns with the natural flow of the universe. This alignment not only enhances our wellbeing but also attracts opportunities, relationships, and experiences that enrich our lives.

Your own circumstances might appear to you like a mountain or hill, insurmountable and vast. It might seem like you are alone dealing with hardship and misfortune.

When we are stuck in our problem, we do not see a way out, we are literally stuck in our own way of thinking and being. Our problem is magnified beyond proportion, we get ourselves frustrated and feel like we are out of options and spinning in circles.

Just this morning, I was getting myself frustrated as I missed the chance to edit my recurring monthly order before the deadline, US customer service wasn't open yet to correct the mistake I made and I was thinking it was too late. My oldest child immediately offered why don't you call European customer service? They're already open. I was glad I followed this advice and the problem was solved, I was able to get on with my day unscathed.

When you cannot help yourself, help others with something. When you help others, the outlook that you have on your problem changes. You suddenly feel good enough, capable enough, courageous enough, you suddenly have the resources and tools to make things happen. The emotional satisfaction you get in exchange is priceless. You vibrate differently, you shift from lack and into abundance, as the saying goes, you cannot give from an empty cup, only from overflow. You start to appreciate the things you took for granted earlier, without having to lose them first. I took walking for granted until I dislocated my knee, now everyday I take my morning walk, I am grateful that I can. I say, thank you my knees for walking. I dislocated my knee three years ago, but I haven't missed a day when I say thanks. The little and great tasks that we do on autopilot are the things that others might find useful. Help yourself by getting out of the microcosm of your problem, help others in the way only you can.

"The more we give away, the more is given to us." – Wayne W. Dyer

---

Every time you help someone, you create a ripple, where your own kindness is passed on to the next person. As the saying goes, you reap what you sow. Giving without expectation of getting anything in return is the best kind of giving, it is untainted and open.

Do you remember a time when you gave something unconditionally?

Why is unconditional love so treasured without pretense or expectation? Sometimes these are not physical things but rather our time and the attention we give.

When raising kids, the most treasured thing is spending time with them, not the physical gifts that we give but the experiences we share with them. My son gets so excited when we watch movies together. He loves doing this daily, sometimes it does not happen due to my busyness, but it is the best quality time together. He also enjoys rock climbing, unfortunately the rock-climbing gym is about an hour away, so going there is an occasion that he enjoys immensely. This morning my older child was awake, and I took her with me to the beach for my morning walk. We enjoyed a cloud-free bright blue sky, a beautiful sunrise, fresh breeze of the ocean and the chirping of birds.

The basic principle of the Law of Attraction is we don't get what we want, we get who we are. We get what we think about, talk about, feel about. If we talk about how everything is bad, we would attract more of that. If we think about illness, we would get more of the same. If we feel we were treated unfairly, betrayed, unworthy, we would get more of that. The point of attraction is what we focus on the most.

If you were to analyze your day, what do you focus on the most?

Do you complain about all the struggles in your life?

Do you find that it is other people's fault as to the state of how you feel?

Do you think that somehow because you talk about this all the time the solution will come to you?

Do you know you are a powerful creator?

You're capable of creating the life you desire but your thoughts, ideas, actions and words have to match and by letting go of past hurts, aches and pains and forgiving who you were. Think of yourself as the musical conductor who is creating your masterpiece.

The other part is the wanting part. The word "want" stems

from lack, meaning something you don't already have. It is a paradox, how can we?

Everything is a vibration, and the word "want" vibrates differently from the word "have".

When we cultivate a mindset of abundance, love, and service, we magnetize experiences and people that reflect these qualities. We human beings are powerful magnets, we attract, magnetize what we think about, what we say and how we feel. So, it is crucial to minimize negative thoughts, feelings and emotions. Of course, life comes with its ups and downs and you are allowed to feel upset, angry, and frustrated, but don't make it your whole life experience. Minimize or limit how long these episodes last.

One great thing I learned from Mahatria is when something negative happens allow yourself one sentence to express it. When something positive occurs, write three sentences about it. Express your joy genuinely, make it significant, make it important, and celebrate yourself! Your life will become better as a result. Remember to eliminate three words from your vocabulary: No, Don't and Not. These three words are bumpers that are preventing you from what you wish to achieve. We constantly create our future, every minute of every day. So, if you set your intentions in the morning and did your meditation practice but continue to practice bad habits of repeating No, Don't and Not, all your great efforts will go to waste.

Become your own best friend and ally instead of your own greatest enemy. Practice saying and thinking beneficial statements. It will take some practice and getting used to, but it is possible to achieve.

Our thoughts, words and actions create our reality whether we want it or not. Every second of every day, whether you are in a good mood or bad, feeling angry, happy, sad or enraged, the magnet of your attention is working. It is up to you what you want to create.

Here is how the Law of Attraction worked in my life. It started with reciting what I wanted to create, what life I wanted to experience. During power hour as dubbed by Tony Robbins back in 2015, I would recite my life story. I wanted to be an author and a writer among many other things. Two years ago in 2022 the dream of becoming an author came true. I didn't know how it would come to pass, but I knew what I wanted. It is pure magic and looking back, if I were to connect the dots, a beautiful constellation will appear, consisting of people I met along the way and the experiences I had that brought me here today.

It started with me going to the Growth Summit in Phoenix, AZ in September 2019. I was inspired by Evan Carmichael, who said there is not enough belief in the world today and you should help somebody who is a step behind you. After all, we all walk each other home. This was the biggest investment of my life to join a mastermind with Brendon Burchard. There I met incredible people who did amazing things. I finally felt that I wasn't crazy. I got a coach who helped me create my first online course. Shortly after, I got inspired by a fellow mastermind member who was doing interviews about people's life journeys. I thought what a great idea!

Wouldn't it be awesome to interview single parents and share their life experiences, challenges and wins? That was how the Single Parent Success Stories podcast started back in 2020. My first guests were fellow mastermind members who believed in my idea and were brave enough to share their stories.

My love for learning kept me going when another mastermind member invited me to attend the challenge framework, led by Pedro Adao. I learned a great deal and discovered an awesome community of heart centered change makers. I met one leader there who ran a series of challenges about finding purpose. He introduced me to another incredible community called the Serving Circle who are all about serving and uplifting the world.

I met a podcaster through that community who then introduced me to the publisher who happened to be a former single mom. I invited her to share her story on my podcast and she invited me to become a contributing author of the Sacred Surrender book. As they say the rest was history. At the time of starting my first podcast I didn't even think it would lead me to becoming an author. I completely forgot about that idea, but the universe remembered and brought it to me as a gift.

Service is a profound expression of love and compassion. When we serve others without expecting anything in return, we become conduits of positive energy, contributing to the collective well-being. This act of selflessness not only uplifts those we serve but also elevates our own spirit, fostering a deep sense of fulfillment and connection.

To fully harness the power of the Law of Attraction through service, it's important to act from a place of genuine love and compassion. When we serve with an open heart, without attachment to specific outcomes, we allow the universe to work its magic. Trusting that our acts of kindness will return to us in unexpected ways is key to attracting abundance.

Practical Steps to Attract Abundance Through Service

Reflect on the skills, talents, and resources you have that can benefit others. Everyone has something valuable to offer, whether it's time, expertise, or simply a listening ear. By identifying your unique gifts, you can find meaningful ways to serve that align with your passions and strengths.

Begin each day by setting an intention to serve others in some way. This could be as simple as offering a smile to a stranger or as significant as volunteering for a cause you care about. Setting this intention primes your mind to look for opportunities to give, which in turn aligns you with the frequency of abundance.

Gratitude is a powerful tool in amplifying the effects of the Law of Attraction. After each act of service, take a moment to express gratitude for the opportunity to give. This reinforces the positive energy you've created and attracts more of it into your life.

Imagine the impact your service has on others and the world around you. Visualizing the ripple effect of your kindness can strengthen your belief in the abundance you're creating, making it more likely to manifest in your own life.

In serving others, we unlock the door to a life filled with abundance, purpose, and joy. By aligning our actions with the principles of the Law of Attraction, we not only enhance the lives of those around us but also invite the universe to shower us with its infinite blessings. The gift inside each of us grows brighter with every act of service, illuminating your path and leading you to a richer, more fulfilling life.

THE GIFT INSIDE

"If you can tune into your purpose and really align with it, setting goals so that your vision is an expression of that purpose, then life flows much more easily." — Jack Canfield

Knowing what you want is key. Sometimes we can spend a lifetime still seeking the answer to that question. Life is a buffet full of experiences to pick and choose from. When encountering a pleasant sensation, feeling or sound or marveling at beauty and wonders of the world, bring these to your joy treasure box. These are the ingredients for your life's recipe. Just like music is made up of individual notes that produce certain sounds, your life is a summation of the experiences and memories and the kind of song you like to sing or dance to. If you were a book what would be the title, what would it be about? If you were a song, would it be happy or sad, noisy and loud or soft and light.

Sometimes we go through life, never asking that question of why am I here? What is my purpose? We don't learn that we can create and just follow and fulfill the expectations of our environment or the dominant voice in our lives, too afraid to break free and cause a ruckus, too afraid to be different for fear we'll be left alone and no one to understand us, no one to guide us. We keep our song to ourselves instead of unleashing it, removing all the masks and being who we truly are. You are unique, you have a gift inside, a purpose and why you are here.

Are you ready to learn what it is?

Do you dare to be different, do you dare to find your true calling?

It is an interesting journey in this game called life. Sometimes we forget and become too serious in deciding what we must do. I would like to invite you to remember how curious you once were about living, learning and playing. I want you to remember that inner child that you have still inside you.

What are the hidden treasures and desires you have?

Have you realized your dreams or are you in pursuit of them?

Have you allowed possibility into your life or are you too concerned with predictability?

Have you connected with the innermost side of who you are or are you too busy living life?

Our time here is limited, it is time to wake up and live your life on your terms. Stop giving in to other people's expectations of who they think you should be and how you should live. Especially people who do not contribute to your well-being, emotionally, mentally or financially.

Engage in practices that foster deep self-reflection and introspection, like journaling, meditation, or spending time in nature.

This will allow you to tune into your inner voice and uncover your true desires and passions. Is there something you wanted to do or be for the longest time but didn't allow yourself to pursue that passion, career, or a great adventure? Through exploring your passions, desires and dreams you uncover a part of yourself that honors your inner voice or higher self.

Explore your values and beliefs to understand what truly matters to you.

Coming into alignment with your core principles will guide you toward a purpose that resonates deeply with your soul. The beliefs you have about the nature of existence, the purpose of life, and our interconnectedness with others and the universe can point us in the right direction. Our values shape our attitudes, behaviors and priorities, guiding us in living authentically and in alignment with what matters most to us. By delving into your inner thoughts and feelings, you can gain insight into what truly matters to you and align your actions with your practices. A simple exercise can involve creating a list and ranking values in order of importance. Then take a moment to reflect on how your current lifestyle aligns with your values.

Some of the common values include honesty, kindness, compassion, freedom and love. Select the ones that resonate deeply with you. Once those are defined, ask yourself these 3 questions:

How can I incorporate these values into my daily life and decision making?

Are there any values that I would like to prioritize more intentionally?

Are there any values that no longer serve me, and if so, how can I let go of them?

"Life is never made unbearable by circumstances, but only by lack of meaning and purpose." — *Viktor Frankl*

Learn to express your true self without fear of judgment.

Embrace your unique strengths and weaknesses, recognizing that authenticity is key to living a purposeful life. How often do you criticize yourself? When a mishap, a mistake or circumstance occurs is your self-critic on high alert?

It is easy to criticize yourself if you were raised by people who constantly strived for perfection. Maybe it is their voice you hear every time you miss a step. I am here to tell you that it is possible to break this unhelpful habit. It takes effort and reinforcement to become the best advocate for yourself. It first starts with becoming aware of your inner critic, followed by reversing and refocusing your attention and then you will be able to see every circumstance as the universe is conspiring for you. It is looking for the silver lining in any situation even if it appears "bad" on the outside.

The judge most likely comes because all your life you were striving to improve your weaknesses, taking strengths for granted as an afterthought. Embracing both sides of the equation balances things out. The world is full of generalists, a mile wide and an inch thick, be a specialist, a mile deep and an inch wide. Be the master by playing on your strengths and work on weaknesses with a gentle heart, like a parent who loves their child with lots of patience and care.

How often do you suppress yourself from being who you are because you want to be accepted and "normal". Whatever "normal" means to you, it is a different thing for different people. When you decide that being "normal" is more important, you rob the world of your quirkiness and uniqueness, you rob the world of the solution that only you can bring. There is no one like you, so start saying yes to being yourself!

Practice vulnerability by sharing your journey with others.

If you've been hiding all your life, sharing your journey might be difficult. We often think that a fancy degree and a college education gives us permission to open our mouths. We totally dismiss our lived experience. Who am I to share, I don't have a PhD, or a major in English literature, English is not even my first language. When you share your journey with others, there are two things that will happen: you could inspire someone into action, and/or find a community of like-minded people. You can build connections based on honesty, where you don't have to pretend to fit in anymore.

Throughout my journey I was able to find such communities where I felt like myself. I got a chance to bloom and soar when the conditions for my growth were well established. This type of environment can support your goals, desires and aspirations. You're encouraged and inspired and pushed outside of your comfort zone to discover your innate abilities, like a diamond that gets slowly chiseled away and turned from an ordinary rock into a precious stone. Who knows what you might discover if you are willing to pursue something you've never done before.

At one point you were young, curious and excited about life, you were meeting it like a great adventure, standing in awe of everything that is.

What got in the way?

Maybe you have forgotten how to play, you started taking things too seriously, and lost your spark in the process.

Maybe you feel lost and have forgotten who you once were before the marriage, and the kids and the career.

Are you ready to remember your hopes and dreams and create your life on purpose?

After all, life is all about redefining, recreating, and constantly evolving into the next version of yourself. Begin by clearly defining what your purpose is. There is a great tool for that called Ikigai. This is a Japanese concept which refers to something that gives a person a sense of purpose, a reason for living. It is the intersection of what you love, what you are good at, what you can be paid for and what the world needs. Through this introspection you might learn a thing or two about yourself. Write down your purpose statement, ensuring it aligns with your core values and beliefs.

"He who has a why to live can bear almost any how." — *Nietzsche*

Transform your purpose into specific, actionable goals.

Divide these goals into manageable steps to avoid feeling over-whelmed. For example, if your purpose involves helping others, set goals related to volunteering, mentoring someone in need, or starting a community project. Integrate your purpose into your daily routine so that you are constantly reminded of your goals. Create rituals or habits, such as a morning intention setting practice or a nightly reflection on your progress.

Make a conscious effort to take daily actions that align with your purpose. Whether big or small, each step should reflect your commitment to living a purposeful life. Consistency builds momentum and reinforces your dedication to redefining who you are. It can be a lonely journey, so finding someone who shares your values and can help hold you accountable would be beneficial. This could be a friend, mentor or coach who supports your journey and provides encouragement and constructive feedback.

I would not be who I am today if it wasn't for my mentors and coaches. My first coach caused me to discover my talents outside of my career and to pay attention to the lived experiences which count for something far greater than a career ever could. Your career is only one aspect of who you are, it is true you spend most of your living life in one career and less so in any other area. But your career does not define you, unless you let it, you are still a person on the inside.

Periodically review your goals and actions to ensure they are still aligned with your purpose. As the saying goes, what you do not measure does not improve. This exercise can help you focus on the task at hand and allow you to track your progress. Sometimes adjustments are necessary to allow for the moving parts. Just like an airplane traveling from point A to point B needs to adjust its course if there is a wind current or other unexpected situation that might occur. You have the power to make adjustments based on other variables as needed to stay on track and remain flexible to adapt to new opportunities that may arise.

Identify ways to serve others that resonate with your purpose. This could involve volunteering for a cause you care about, sharing your skills and knowledge with those in need, or simply offering support and kindness to those around you. Take a look at all the activities that you do and you may find that it is already happening. Giving back offers you an opportunity to share what you are best at and allows others to receive that help.

Look for opportunities to create a positive impact in your community or beyond. This could be accomplished through starting initiatives, participating in local events, or using your talents to address societal issues. The act of giving back not only benefits others but it also deepens your sense of fulfillment and connection to your purpose.

Take time to reflect on how your actions are making a difference.

I am blessed and grateful to create space for people to share their stories through speaking and writing. Giving single parents and women hope to know there is light in the end of the tunnel. Life is possible and beautiful after the darkest of clouds and if I can do it, you can too!

Acknowledge the positive impact you are creating and celebrate your achievements. Celebrating your wins lets your mind know why you do what you do and reinvigorates you to keep going.

I invite you to keep going, keep discovering the gift that you are by creating a practice based on the tools that I have shared in this book.

THE JOURNEY AHEAD

*C*ongratulations on completing this book!

Here are a few ideas for your to consider:

1. If you haven't emailed your receipt or a picture of you with the book yet, send it to support@irinashehovsov.com to get your *free bonuses*.

2. I'd love to have your help spreading the message. If you read the book, **please consider sharing** it with your friends and online so that more people can learn the wisdom that is essential but not taught in schools. If you create any videos or posts, tag me in them. I'd love to see what you thought of the book and how it is helping you.

3. If you received great value from the book, consider buying a copy for a friend. If it made a meaningful difference for you,

it'll make a meaningful difference for others and **you will be remembered** as a person who introduced them to it.

4. Most importantly, **take action**. Don't let this book just sit on your shelf and collect dust. Do something. You don't get changes in your life by reading, you get them by taking action.
I can't wait to see and hear about your progress. I'm honored to be a guide on your happiness journey.
Love,
Irina

REFLECTING ON YOUR TRANSFORMATION

Recapping the 12 Steps: Your Journey of Growth

A Holistic Review: Take a moment to revisit the 12 steps you've undertaken—each chapter represents a significant milestone on your path to rediscovering happiness. Reflect on how each step has influenced your physical, emotional, mental, and spiritual well-being. Get curious about your happiness journey and seek to improve it through practicing the 12 steps:

1. Create a morning routine that suits you, how you want to wake up, what are the things that get you going, what would be the best start to your day?

2. Improve your eating habits – choose whole foods over processed foods, examine your hydration habits and make improvements where necessary.

3. Move – so you can sustain focus, effort and wellbeing, add energy to your day and move your emotions from stagnation into action.

4. Meditate – remember to take the inner shower for the mind, to create clarity, presence and ease for your day.

5. Pursue your passions – it is never too late to practice your hobbies. No matter your age or position in life, do what makes you happy.

6. Be present – be present in your life, let future and past be gone, be here and now. Experience and fully take in your life.

7. Become free from victimhood – accept responsibility for your life, look for lessons from the experience rather than punishment and let go of the past.

8. Deal with overwhelm – prioritize your life, create a routine, practice stress relief on a regular basis and speak good things unto you.

9. Environment – what kind of people are you surrounded by? Do they add or subtract from your life? Make sure to create a positive circle of people who see more in you than you see in yourself.

10. Be Happy Now – it is up to you to decide to be happy. It is not hidden outside of you, it is always on the inside. Just like an electric plant generates electricity, you can generate happiness from within.

11. Serve Others – whatever is your magic, share it with others and help in your own unique way.

12. The Gift Inside – discover your purpose and share it with the world

These are the twelve steps that can support you to create your happiness and stay there. These are the habits that will make you feel alive, be more present, appreciate the journey and be happy.

So what now? Keep this checklist of the twelve habits with you at all times. You can find a summary guide at the end of the book. If you'd like to continue your research and learning in this area, consider joining the Happiness Academy program.

When you are ready visit: https://www.irinashehovsov.com/https://www.irinashehovsov.com

Nine years ago, I stood out of breath and exhausted after missing my train to work by a second. I learned that life is not about constant suffering and happiness is possible only if we let ourselves have it. I didn't particularly like where I was, so I sought to change my life and looked for ways to make it better. I didn't want to live a life of regret, I wanted to find happiness. Live, dream and grow became my mantra. That striving led to a life of learning and ultimately, to the discovery of these twelve steps.

I hope that as you close this book, you decide to live with similar intentions and reinvent your life. I hope you wake up each day and decide to practice these steps that will make you content with your life. I hope that as you endeavor to live a happy life, you pursue your passions, let go of the past, and find your gift. Your happiness is an inside job and you too have the gift inside.

SUMMARY GUIDE

PHYSICAL HEALTH

Step one: Morning Routine

1. _Establish a Morning Routine_ Create a routine that makes you feel alive each morning. A structured morning routine sets a positive tone for the day, helping you feel more grounded and in control. Start by waking up 30 minutes earlier than usual. Use this time to engage in activities like walking, meditation, stretching, or journaling. Gradually build up your routine by adding one new habit each week, such as reading or practicing mindfulness. Make sure to include elements to awaken your body, mind and soul.

Check out peaceful warrior routine at https://www.irinashe-hovsov.com/tgi

2. _Practice Mindful Walking_ Walking, especially in the morning, can clear your mind, improve mood, and increase your physical energy. Begin with a 20-30 minutes walk each morning. As you walk, focus on your surroundings, observe the colors of the sky, the scent of the air, and feel the wind on your face. This practice helps you stay present and appreciate the small joys of life.

3. _Incorporate Positive Affirmations_ Speaking life into yourself can reshape your mindset, boost self-confidence, and inspire you to take action toward your goals. During your morning routine, dedicate time to visualize your ideal life. Speak positive affirmations aloud, such as "I am capable," "I am worthy," or "I am creating the life I desire." Envision your future successes and feel the emotions associated with achieving them.

Step two: Healthy Eating

1. _Incorporate Whole Foods Gradually_ Start by making small changes to your diet, like replacing processed snacks with whole foods such as fresh fruits, vegetables, nuts, and seeds. Over time, these small shifts will lead to a more nourishing and balanced diet that supports both physical and mental well-being. Check out Holobowl recipe at https://www.irinashe-hovsov.com/tgi

2. _Practice Mindful Eating_ Engage in mindful eating by paying full attention to the taste, texture, and aroma of your food. This practice not only enhances your eating experience but

also helps you tune into your body's hunger and fullness cues, reducing the likelihood of overeating or emotional eating.

3. _Prioritize Hydration_ Make hydration a daily priority by aiming to drink at least 8 glasses of water a day. Consider adding water-rich foods like cucumbers and melons to your diet, and try incorporating herbal teas or broths for additional hydration and nutrients. This simple habit can significantly improve your physical and mental clarity.

Step three: Movement

1. _Integrate Movement into Your Daily Routine_ Start by making small changes in your daily habits, such as choosing stairs over elevators and setting a timer to remind yourself to stand and walk every hour. These small adjustments can significantly improve cardiovascular health, increase leg strength, and maintain energy levels throughout the day. Your body was designed to move. Move like your life depends on it.

2. _Adopt a Simple, Sustainable Workout Routine_ Incorporate a minimal yet effective workout routine like the 10x training program, which requires only 15 minutes of exercise twice a week, focusing on major muscle groups. This approach makes it easier to maintain consistency without the need for extensive gym time, leading to increased strength, reduced body fat, and improved overall well-being. Infuse movement into your day, a little bit at a time. Introduce exercise snacks and short movement bursts throughout your day.

Check out a sample 10x fitness routine at https://www.iri-nashehovsov.com/tgi

3. _Prioritize Sleep and Recovery_ Establish a calming evening routine to improve sleep quality. This includes cutting off electronics two hours before bed, taking your last meal four hours before sleep, and creating a sleep-friendly environment (dark, cool room). Quality sleep enhances physical recovery, boosts mental clarity, and increases resilience, contributing to better overall health and peace of mind.

EMOTIONAL HEALTH

Step four: Meditation

1. _Create a Dedicated Meditation Space_ Set aside a specific area in your home where you can meditate regularly. This space should be quiet, comfortable, and free from distractions. Personalize it with a cushion, blanket, or any items that bring you peace, such as candles or crystals. The consistency of using the same space will help anchor your practice and make it easier to enter a meditative state.

2. _Establish a Daily Morning Meditation Routine_ Begin your day with a short meditation practice, even if it's just 5-10 minutes. This can be a simple mindfulness meditation where you focus on your breath, or a guided meditation that centers on themes like forgiveness or gratitude. Starting your day with meditation helps clear your mind, set a positive tone, and prepare you to face the day with clarity and calmness.

3. *Practice Forgiveness and Gratitude Meditation* Incorporate specific meditations focused on forgiveness and gratitude into your routine. Spend a few minutes each day visualizing the release of anger, resentment, and past hurts. Follow this with a gratitude meditation where you acknowledge and appreciate the positive aspects of your life, no matter how small. Over time, this practice will shift your mindset, helping you to let go of past traumas and cultivate a more positive, resilient outlook on life.

Check out a self-love meditation at https://www.irinashe-hovsov.com/tgi

Step five: Hobbies

1. *Explore New Interests Regularly* Dedicate time each month to trying something new. This could be as simple as tasting a new cuisine, picking up a new book genre, or attending a workshop or class that piques your interest. Constantly seeking out new experiences keeps life exciting, stimulates your mind and can lead to discovering hidden talents or passions. Pursue your passions, don't wait for better days to come.

2. *Incorporate a Creative Hobby into Your Routine* Choose a hobby that excites you, whether it's painting, writing, dancing, or music, and commit to practicing it regularly—at least once a week. Join a local club or group to stay motivated. Engaging in a hobby allows you to unwind, tap into your creative side and brings a sense of accomplishment and joy, which can enhance your overall well-being.

3. _Push Beyond Your Comfort Zone_ Identify something that scares or challenges you, like public speaking, performing, or learning a difficult skill and take the first step toward conquering it. Set small, achievable goals to build confidence. Pushing yourself to face fears or trying challenging activities builds resilience, boosts confidence, and opens up new opportunities for personal growth and fulfillment.

Step six: Being Present

1. _Engage Fully with Your Senses in Nature_ Next time you are outdoors, consciously remove all distractions like your phone or other devices. Tune into the environment using all your senses: listen to the sounds around you, feel the wind against your skin, observe the shapes and colors of your surroundings, smell and taste the air as you breathe deeply. This practice helps you ground yourself in the present moment, allowing you to fully experience life as it happens, rather than being caught up in past regrets or future worries. Savor each moment of life.

2. _Practice Mindful Hugging_ When you hug someone, focus entirely on that moment. Let go of thoughts about your to-do lists or other distractions. Instead notice how your body feels, how the other person's warmth and presence affect you, and how your breath slows down. This simple yet profound practice can reduce stress, increase feelings of safety and connection, and remind you to cherish the small, meaningful moments that make up your life.

3. _Set Daily Reminders for Mindfulness_ Set daily reminders on

your phone with a message like "You are enough" or "You have a lot in your life to be grateful for, Be present, Stay happy, You are loved". When the reminder goes off, take a moment to stop whatever you're doing and bring your attention to the present. Reflect on the message and what it means to you. This consistent practice helps build the habit of mindfulness, training your brain to focus on the present moment, which can reduce your anxiety and increase overall well-being.

MENTAL HEALTH

Step seven: Becoming Free From Victimhood

1. *Take Personal Responsibility* Reflect on the choices and actions that have led to your current situation. Acknowledge that while external circumstances can be challenging, your response and decisions play a crucial role in shaping your reality. Start a daily journal and record situations where you feel powerless. Then, identify at least one way you could have influenced the outcome. Over time, this practice will help you recognize patterns and areas where you can take more control.

2. *Shift Your Focus from Problem to Solution* Instead of dwelling on what is wrong or broken, actively seek out solutions. Shift your mindset from "Why did this happen to me?" to "What can I learn from this?" For every challenge you face, write down at least three potential solutions or lessons. Commit to taking one actionable step toward resolving the issue and learning from it.

3. _Practice Observing, Not Absorbing_ Develop the habit of viewing your life experiences objectively, as if you were an observer or scientist studying the situation. This detachment allows you to learn from your experiences without being emotionally overwhelmed. When confronted with a negative experience, take a few moments to breathe deeply and mentally step back. Ask yourself, "What can I observe here without judgment?" Practice this regularly to build emotional resilience and clarity.

Step eight: Dealing with Overwhelm

1. _Prioritize and Manage Time Effectively_ Break down overwhelming tasks into smaller, manageable steps. Start by identifying the top three most critical tasks for the day. Focus on completing these before moving on to less urgent tasks. Time blocking can also help, where you allocate specific blocks of time to different tasks, ensuring that you stay on track and maintain a balanced schedule.

2. _Practice Stress Reduction Techniques_ Incorporate stress-reducing activities into your daily routine. This could include taking short breaks to change your physical state, such as stretching, walking, or engaging in deep breathing exercises. Additionally, consider reframing negative thoughts by practicing mindfulness or using positive affirmations to shift your mindset.

3. _Set Boundaries and Learn to Say No_ Protect your mental and emotional health by setting clear boundaries. This might involve saying no to additional responsibilities that could lead

to burnout or overwhelm. Focus on what truly matters and delegate tasks when possible, to prevent spreading yourself too thin. By respecting your limits, you create space for self-care and recovery, which is essential for long-term well-being.

Step nine: Your Environment

1. _Create a Vision and Use Affirmations_ Draft a clear vision of who you want to become, writing it as if you already possess these qualities. Recite the vision daily, particularly in the morning and evening, when your mind is more receptive. This practice will help rewire your subconscious mind, reinforcing your desired identity.

2. _Curate Your Environment_ Identify and consciously choose to spend time in environments and with people who uplift and inspire you. Whether it's a supportive community, engaging in hobbies, or simply being around positive individuals, curating your surroundings to reflect your desired growth will help foster the traits you aspire to develop. Examine your environment. Is it draining or uplifting?

3. _Stay Open and Curious_ Embrace a beginner's mindset and remain open to new possibilities and experiences. Engage in activities that spark curiosity and challenge your current perspectives. This openness will allow you to continually grow and adapt, keeping your mindset flexible and resilient.

SPIRITUAL HEALTH

Step ten: Be Happy Now

1. _Define and Pursue Your Personal Happiness_ Define what happiness means to you. Write it down in detail–what it looks like, feels like, and sounds like. Consider your perfect day and the small moments that bring you joy. Start by listing three things that genuinely make you happy, whether it's a daily habit or an activity. Incorporate these into your daily routine, no matter how small they are.

2. _Practice Gratitude Daily_ Shift your focus from what's wrong to what's going right. Each day, consciously practice gratitude, especially during challenging moments. Keep a daily gratitude journal. Every night, write down three things you are grateful for, focusing on small, often overlooked moments that brought you joy and peace. We cannot control the circumstances, but we do control how we react to them. At the end of the day, life is 20% what happens and 80% how you react to what happens.

3. _Cultivate Mindfulness and Presence_ Make a conscious effort to be present in your daily life, noticing the small, beautiful moments that often go unnoticed. Practice mindfulness through simple activities like deep breathing, observing nature, or savoring your meals. Set aside 5-10 minutes each day to be fully present, appreciating the moment without distractions.

Step eleven: Serving Others

1. _Identify and Offer Your Unique Gifts:_ Reflect on the skills, talents, and resources you possess that can benefit others. Whether it's your time, expertise, or simply being a good listener, everyone has something valuable to offer. Start by identifying these gifts and look for ways to share them with those in need. This can be as simple as helping a neighbor or volunteering for a cause that aligns with your passions. By doing so, you align yourself with the energy of abundance and create opportunities for positive experiences to flow into your life.

2. _Set a Daily Intention to Serve:_ Begin each day with the intention to serve others in some capacity. This doesn't have to be a grand gesture; it could be as small as offering a kind word to a colleague or lending a hand to a friend. By consciously deciding to serve, you prime your mind to seek out opportunities to give, which in turn aligns you with the frequency of abundance. This simple practice can transform your mindset and attract more positivity into your life.

3. _Practice Gratitude After Each Act of Service:_ After every act of service, take a moment to express gratitude for the opportunity to give. This not only reinforces the positive energy you've created but also amplifies the effects of the Law of Attraction. By being grateful, you attract more of the same energy into your life, opening the door to further abundance and joy. This simple practice can transform your mindset and attract more positivity into your life.

Step twelve: The Gift Inside

1. *Discover and Embrace Your True Self*: Start by dedicating time each day to introspective practices like journaling, meditation, or spending time in nature. These activities help you tune into your inner voice and uncover your true desires and passions. Set aside at least 10-15 minutes daily for journaling or meditation, focusing on what brings you joy and fulfillment. Write down any insights or feelings that arise during this time.

2. *Identify and Prioritize Your Core Values:* Reflect on your values and beliefs to understand what truly matters to you. This will guide you toward a purpose that aligns with your authentic self. Create a list of your core values, rank them in order of importance, and assess how your current lifestyle aligns with these values. Then, take one small action daily to better align your life with your top values.

3. *Transform Purpose into Actionable Goals:* Clearly identify your purpose and break it down into specific, manageable goals that align with your values and passions. Integrate these goals into your daily routine to stay focused and motivated. Then, break it down into three actionable goals. Begin incorporating these goals into your daily life, starting with small, consistent steps.

These twelve habits and practices will allow you to craft your own path to happiness. There are other basic strategies in the book but these twelve are the ones that will create the breakthrough you seek. For even more resources, including checklists, posters, daily planners, journals and training tools, visit https://www.irinashehovsov.com/tgi

ABOUT THE AUTHOR

IRINA SHEHOVSOV

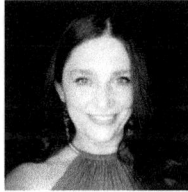

Irina Shehovsov is the Founder of Reclaim Your Life, trans-formational coach and 5x #1 International Best-Selling Author. She believes that, just like an electric plant generates electricity, you can generate happiness from within. She stands by these three words, Live, Dream and Grow. Living is about wellness of physical, mental, emotional and spiritual states of being. Dreaming is about the pursuit of dreams. Growing is about continuous evolution and growth as we learn about ourselves and the world around us and make it a better place for the future. She is the host of two podcasts Single Parent Success Stories and Reclaim Your Life with Irina and runs a YouTube channel called Happiness Academy. Irina's intention is to empower women to believe in them-selves, no matter what anyone says.